Advance praise for
The Neurogenesis Diet and Lifestyle

THE NEUROGENESIS
DIET AND LIFESTYLE

THE
NEUROGENESIS
DIET AND LIFESTYLE

UPGRADE YOUR BRAIN, UPGRADE YOUR LIFE

BRANT CORTRIGHT, PH.D.

PSYCHE MEDIA

Cover Design: Derek Murphy
Copyeditor: Madeline Hopkins
Inside Design: Jake Muelle

Published by:
Psyche Media
55 Millside Lane
Mill Valley, CA

PSYCHE MEDIA

This book is for educational purposes only. If you know or suspect you have a health problem, you should consult a health professional. The author and publisher specifically disclaim any liability, loss, or risk, personal or otherwise, that is incurred as a consequence, directly or indirectly, of the use and application of any of the contents of this book.

ISBN: 978-0-9861492-0-7

CONTENTS

CHAPTER 1

THE NEUROGENESIS REVOLUTION

Your life can be so much more than it is now. Imagine having increased energy, a better memory, and starting each day feeling positive and rested, ready to tackle whatever challenges may come. Recent advances in medical science have put this goal within reach. **You and everyone you know has a vast, untapped potential to live more fully.** But to realize your greatest potential your brain must operate at its highest level.

The key to tapping this potential is **neurogenesis,** the process of creating new neurons, or brain cells. **Neurogenesis is how the brain renews and upgrades itself.**

Understanding neurogenesis is the most revolutionary discovery of neuroscience in the past century. Although there is still much to be learned, recent studies have revealed that the process can be enhanced and encouraged by individual lifestyle choices. **To increase neurogenesis is to improve your entire life— how you think, feel, and act.**

Research shows that high rates of neurogenesis are associated with:

- higher cognitive function
- better memory and faster learning
- emotional vitality and resilience
- protection from stress, anxiety, and depression
- elevated immunity
- enhanced overall brain function

Increasing neurogenesis dramatically improves everyday life at all stages and radically transforms what aging looks and feels like.

This is the first book that tells you what you can do to effect these changes in your own life. Never before has this information been gathered together and presented in one place.

Remember a time when you were at the top of your game—confident, flowing, articulate, expansive, knowing what needed to be done and doing it. If difficulties arose you knew you could overcome them and bounce back. **Now imagine feeling this way every day.** Maybe not 100% of the time, but imagine living at a higher level and feeling on top of it, solid in yourself, the vast majority of the time. That's what this book intends to bring about.

Several years have gone into researching this book, combing, compiling, and correlating the neuroscience research literature to cohesively present vital information that was scattered in obscure technical journals. **This is the most important news for brain health and human life in recent history.** It will revolutionize the way you look at aging and the choices you make in your daily life. No longer do you need to passively submit to a middle-age decline in brain function, then a further decline in old age. You will never be "over the hill" because there is no hill and never was, only a constant, steady progression. But with this book you can even *increase* your rate of neurogenesis—in your twenties, thirties, middle or old age—and consequently upgrade your brain and your life.

At any age, you can operate at a higher level than has ever before been possible.

The Neurogenesis Revolution in Brain Science

With this in mind, let's look at five major breakthroughs, or paradigm shifts, in neuroscience that revolutionize how we see the brain.

Breakthrough #1 – The brain keeps growing new brain cells your entire life. This process of neurogenesis is how the brain upgrades itself and enhances your quality of life.

To recap the last century of brain science, up until the late 1990s neuroscience accepted as fact that the brain stops growing new brain cells by adulthood. It was believed that after this cessation, it was just one slow, unavoidable slide into decrepitude as brain cells die off, never to be replaced, gradually at first, but then faster and faster as you age. **Then scientists discovered this is all wrong.** So what changed?

In the 1950s medical science found out that the brain is more malleable, adaptable, and fluid than had been previously thought. This neural plasticity allows the brain to make new connections among neurons and to heal, to some degree, after traumatic brain injuries or strokes. Then in recent decades we learned that the brain's adaptability and plasticity are even greater than at first suspected.

In the 1980s and '90s, as neuroscience technology developed better instruments to measure the brain, more evidence emerged from various researchers pointing to new neurons being formed in the hippocampus of other adult mammals.

It had long been known that the hippocampus is involved in forming new memories and plays a critical role in reasoning and remembering. **Damage to the hippocampus results in cognitive deficits and memory problems.** This has been proven by countless studies and research into related injuries and illnesses. Alzheimer's disease, for example, massively attacks the hippocampus, as do other kinds of dementia.

The ability to create new memories—which we do throughout our lives—means something new is happening in the brain, suggesting some kind of plasticity or dynamism. This insight plus the recently realized possibility of adult neurogenesis led pioneering neuroscientist Fred Gage, Ph.D., of the Salk Institute in San Diego, to explore the hippocampus in a new way. [1] In the late 1990s Gage showed definitively that, contrary to almost a century of accepted wisdom, adult human brains do indeed create new brain cells. [2] This groundbreaking discovery has since been confirmed many times over.

Gage's findings shook the foundations of everything science thought it knew about the brain.

It instantly exploded two myths about the brain and aging that had been unquestioned "facts" before this.

Myth – Your brain stops growing in your early twenties. After that you only lose brain cells.

> **Myth** – Aging means cognitive decline and memory loss; after middle age life is just one gradual downhill slide into decrepitude.

The discovery that your brain produces new brain cells as long as you are alive upends the belief that the brain stops growing in young adulthood. It also changes our entire picture of aging, for if new brain cells are being formed, then the brain can renew itself. What is key is **the rate at which new brain cells form.**

> **Breakthrough #2** – There is great variation in people's **rate of neurogenesis.**

People show enormous variation in how high or low their rate of neurogenesis is. Some people's brains create new neurons at a rapid clip, while most people chug along at about the average rate. Still others produce new brain cells at one-fifth the average rate.

There are vast differences in how quickly people produce new brain cells and your rate of neurogenesis may be the single most important factor for a high quality of life. **When neurogenesis is high, you are alive, engaged, expansive, fulfilling your potential.** Your mind's abilities are enhanced and your emotional vitality is strong. You are protected from stress and depression. You feel good and life is fulfilling. Immunity is robust. Your spirits are high and your outlook is positive.

With a low rate of neurogenesis, your brain shrinks, your life contracts, and you move toward memory loss, cognitive deficits, dementia, stress and anxiety, depression, reduced executive function, immunity, and myriad health problems. **When neurogenesis is low your whole quality of life suffers.** Having a high level of neurogenesis may be the most important thing you can do to cultivate a high quality of life.

Your Quality of Life Depends on the Quality of Your Brain

High brain quality doesn't mean high I.Q. or artistic skill or some other talent, rather it means how dynamic, alive, moving, growing your brain is. A high rate of neurogenesis, the creation of new neurons, gives a youthful vitality to the brain.

Breakthrough #3 – Your rate of neurogenesis is tied to the quality of your life.

The quality of your life is directly proportional to your rate of neurogenesis. High rates of neurogenesis confer strong cognitive, emotional, and physical advantages. Conversely, in study after study, reduced neurogenesis is associated with lower cognitive function; memory problems; vulnerability to stress, anxiety, and depression; emotional instability; and overall cognitive deficits. [5-8]

In other words, the research clearly shows:

- A high rate of neurogenesis and you are doing exceedingly well.
- A normal rate of neurogenesis and you are okay, normal, average.

- A low rate of neurogenesis and you're struggling with anxiety, stress, depression, lowered health and immunity, memory problems and cognitive deficits. You are not doing so well.

Broadly speaking we can call anything that nourishes the brain and increases neurogenesis *neurohealthy*, whereas those things that hurt the brain and decrease neurogenesis can be considered *neurotoxic*. **What we believe to be "normal aging" is actually an artifact of a neurotoxic lifestyle that slows the brain down much more and much faster than necessary.**

Usually neurogenesis slows down and plateaus in middle age. Then it decreases even further in old age. However, this doesn't need to be the case. **Neuroscientists recently discovered that neurogenesis can be increased at all ages through proper stimulation.** In fact, it can increase dramatically, with major boosts in cognition, mood, and health.

Although its potential, possibility, and function are just starting to be identified, the rate of neurogenesis could likely be a biological indicator, or biomarker, for overall brain function and even emotional and physical health.[13] Your rate of neurogenesis appears to be not only a biomarker of cognitive health, stress, and depression but perhaps even heart health, since our brain and cardiovascular system are so closely linked.

Breakthrough Science for Brain Enhancement

The discovery that new brain cells can be, and are, constantly created has revolutionized our understanding of the brain. This is not just about extending the brain's best years but actually *enhancing the brain*. This is something we never knew was possible until now.

> **Breakthrough #4** – You can increase your rate of neurogenesis by three to five times at all ages—young, middle-aged, old. You can operate at a higher level of brain function in your twenties and thirties, in middle age as well as your sixties, seventies, and beyond.

You can improve your brain's aliveness and memory. Old age does not have to mean steep decline. **The decay in quality of life, memory, and emotional resilience usually associated with aging is really only a side effect of a neurotoxic lifestyle and diet.** It doesn't need to be this way.

> **Myth** – Your genes determine how you age and how long your brain stays sharp.

> **Myth** – You reach your mental peak in your twenties and thirties. Nothing can be done to make you sharper once you're middle-aged or beyond.

We now know that diet and lifestyle factors significantly outweigh our genetic inheritance. Because these discoveries are so new, the upper limits of successful aging are unknown. We simply don't yet know all that's possible!

An Experiment that Changed the World

In the first few years after neurogenesis was discovered, researchers tried to find out if it was possible to "jump start" the process, to increase the rate at which new neurons form. Dr. Fred Gage gave mice an "enriched environment," consisting of running wheels, areas to explore, nesting materials, other mice to interact and mate with, sensory novelty and complexity, then monitored the effects. The results startled Gage and his team. **Giving mice an "enriched environment" increased neurogenesis by four or five times.** [10]

The part of the brain in which new brain cells can form went from containing 300,000 brain cells to 350,000, an increase of 50,000 neurons. **This is one-sixth more brain cells than in normal mice.**

Perhaps even more surprising than the sheer rate of increase was the powerful effect this had on the abilities of these mice. **The mice with these new brain cells were found to have strongly enhanced cognitive abilities and memory compared to their "normal neurogenesis" peers.** They remembered better, they figured things out faster, they displayed superior all around cognitive abilities. In other words, they were smarter.

Further, these mice developed much greater emotional resources. They were protected from emotional stresses. This protection wasn't absolute, of course, but they had dramatically improved resistance to fear, stress, and depression. **It may be too much to call them "super-mice," but their abilities were significantly enhanced.** Both cognitively and emotionally they had a considerable advantage over their normal peers.

Another unexpected finding was the consistency of the results for mice of different ages. **When this enriched environment began in middle age, there was a five-fold increase in the rate of neurogenesis and** [1, 10] **when it began in old age there was a three- to five-fold increase.** [11, 14]

What was even more surprising about these results was the importance of enriching the environment in many different ways. In normal conditions, 60–70% of new neurons die off, but the enriched environment allowed almost all of the new neurons to survive and develop. **It was the complete lifestyle change, not just one "thing," that yielded such powerful results.**

Reproducing the Results

This experiment has been successfully reproduced many times by other researchers. Further, neuroscientists have broken down the enriched environment to determine what particular effects different environmental stimuli have on neurogenesis. Some things, like certain kinds of exercise, increase the production of new brain cells while others, such as sensory novelty, seem to prevent new cells from being pruned or dying off.

While these exciting findings have pointed to a whole new direction for brain development and aging, the data are so new that neuroscientists have yet to fully explore their significance. **We don't know what optimal childhood, adolescence, or young adulthood looks like.** No one has ever before accelerated neurogenesis in childhood or in young adulthood.

We don't know what optimal middle age looks like. Until recently it wasn't known that neurogenesis even existed, let alone that it slows down in middle age or that it can be accelerated.

Similarly, we don't yet know what optimal old age looks like! But we do know that you can extend your brain health throughout your lifespan, well into your eighties and nineties (and hopefully beyond.)

This information is brand new and the positive effect it can have on aging has yet to be fully observed. Furthermore, because a mother's diet and lifestyle affect her newborn baby's rate of neurogenesis, it will be over a hundred years before we find the upper limits of what's possible in successful aging. **We are in the midst of a brain revolution that even our children won't see the end of.**

What will enhanced primary years and adolescence look like? What will enhanced twenties or thirties look like? What will enhanced middle age and old age look like? We're about to see. **Only now, at this moment in history, can we say how to increase neurogenesis to produce a better, smarter, healthier, more emotionally resilient brain.**

But these results are far from definitive, more information is being uncovered at an astounding rate. Since the discovery of the neurogenesis-boosting effects of an enriched environment, many new nutrients and other factors have also been shown to increase neurogenesis. What effects will this have in further enriching the environment? Will following the program in this book boost neurogenesis eight or ten times normal in optimal conditions? 20 times? We simply don't yet know, as science lags behind this recent research.

But as the research advances and people choose to enhance their rate of neurogenesis by altering their lifestyles, the entire planet will go through a cognitive and emotional boost. As ever larger numbers learn about and adopt the strategies in this book to increase neurogenesis, you may be putting yourself at a cognitive disadvantage by not utilizing these discoveries to realize your brain's full potential.

It looks like the best is yet to come, for all of us. One thing is clear: at any time, you can start to profoundly affect your brain and your life. You can't begin too early—or too late.

Exploding the Myth of Serotonin Deficiency in Depression

What really turned the spotlight on the hippocampus and neurogenesis came almost serendipitously from an entirely different direction in research. **It was the discovery that depression is linked to lowered neurogenesis.**

In 2000 the Yale researcher Jessica Malberg, Ph.D., was researching the neural effects of antidepressants. Quite unexpectedly, she discovered that a class of antidepressant medications called selective serotonin reuptake inhibitors (SSRIs, such as Prozac) increase neurogenesis. [4] This set off a whole new line of thinking about depression. **Maybe neurogenesis, not serotonin, is the key to treating depression.**

Up until then the popular idea was that a "serotonin deficiency" created depression and SSRI medications like Prozac corrected the deficiency. The SSRI class of antidepressants had taken modern bio-psychiatry by storm. At the time of Malberg's discovery, SSRIs were the second most widely prescribed class of medication in the world. **By 2013 SSRIs generated over $15 billion of revenue for the big drug companies.**

Even though SSRIs are effective for less than 50% of patients and frequently have undesirable side effects, such as loss of sexual desire in most patients, Prozac and its cousins (including Celexa, Zoloft, Paxil and Lexapro) quickly became thought of as the greatest thing since sliced bread for psychiatry and the biological theory of depression. **But Malberg's study threatened to undermine the entire "serotonin deficiency" theory.**

Building on Malberg's work and researching people's serotonin levels seemed to undercut the "serotonin deficiency" theory, and by the early 2000s, it was under assault from many quarters. Only a few studies had shown lower serotonin levels in depressed patients, whereas most of the studies showed depressed patients to have either normal or even higher serotonin levels. Additionally, when serotonin levels were lowered experimentally in test subjects, almost no one became depressed or experienced any difference at all in mood.

Plus, a new generation of antidepressants came out that didn't involve serotonin at all but were just as effective, norepinephrine reuptake inhibitors (NRIs) and norepinephrine dopamine reuptake inhibitors (NDRIs). This seemed to debunk the "serotonin deficiency" theory. After all, why would they have any effect on depression if they didn't affect serotonin levels?

Then in 2003 two key data points converged that shifted serotonin from a primary role in depression to being only a minor player. The first was the observation that when patients begin taking an SSRI, their serotonin levels increase dramatically within a few hours. But there is usually no change in mood for three or four weeks. If lack of serotonin is central, shouldn't this affect mood immediately? It turns out that this lag time of three or four weeks is how long it takes new brain cells to become mature, functioning neurons. **This points to neurogenesis as the central mechanism of SSRIs.**

> **Myth** – Depression is a biological illness caused by low serotonin levels. It requires lifelong SSRI drugs to treat it.

The second data point came from a seminal study at the Columbia University lab of Rene Hen, Ph.D. A postdoctoral researcher named Luca Santarelli, Ph.D., gave depressed mice an SSRI to increase serotonin but prevented neurogenesis from occurring. There was no change in depression levels. **This study, since replicated, showed that antidepressants don't work without neurogenesis.** [3] Only when neurogenesis increased did the depression lift. It also explained why NDRIs and NRIs work as antidepressants, since they also increase neurogenesis.

Thus the "serotonin deficiency" theory crumbled as dozens of follow-up studies showed neurogenesis to be the key player in depression. Serotonin is but one of over twenty neurotransmitters that affect mood and emotion. "Serotonin deficiency" was an overly simplistic theory to begin with, but this very simplicity is what made it so appealing and marketable. Now, however, the tide has shifted to a more complex understanding of depression, one in which the rate of neurogenesis is critical.

The increased research into the causes and treatment of depression brought the spotlight onto neurogenesis and the hippocampus. As neurogenesis came into focus through a host of studies, it became clear that a person's rate of neurogenesis is of immense importance for every part of life.

"A Fountain of Youth for the Brain"

For most people the rate of neurogenesis decreases by ages 30–35. In many people it decreases so dramatically that by 40 or 50 or 60 there are noticeable mental effects. **When neurogenesis drops, quality of life goes downhill quickly.** Along with reduced neurogenesis we see such things as:

- memory loss
- cognitive impairments
- chronic stress, anxiety, and fear
- depression

- loss of emotional resilience, trauma
- reduced immunity, chronic illnesses
- diminished executive function
- loss of vitality, lassitude
- dementia

In the adult brain of mammals, new brain cells are formed in two specific regions: the olfactory bulb that registers smells and the hippocampus, an area responsible for forming new memories (cognition), orienting the body in space (sensing), and regulating mood (emotion). It's the hippocampus that holds the key to brain enhancement.

> **Breakthrough #5** – You can operate at a higher level than ever before believed possible. At any age you can be smarter, remember more, be more vibrant, alive, free of depression, and resistant to stress. When you increase your rate of neurogenesis, the farther reaches of the brain's potential is unknown.

So-called normal aging is a by-product of accumulated neurotoxins that reduce neurogenesis. Neurotoxic vs. neurohealthy aging is the difference between night and day. New research indicates the brain can renew itself at any age, and neurogenesis is the very source of renewal for the brain. **Your rate of neurogenesis is key to feeling good or bad, vibrant and rejuvenated or stagnant and depressed.**

We now know there are things you can do to stimulate neurogenesis—at any time in your life. For the first time in the history of the planet, we've discovered that you can increase your rate of neurogenesis by the choices you make in daily life.

A rise in neurogenesis will protect against stress, anxiety, and depression while enhancing cognitive function and learning. Your rate of neurogenesis is a key indicator of quality of life.

How Your Brain Relates to the World Determines Everything

As we have seen, when mice were given an impoverished environment, one that was stressful or barren or isolated, neurogenesis slowed to a crawl and the results were depression, lethargy, fear, activated stress circuits, lack of exploratory behavior, reduced immunity, lack of interest in pleasurable activities, cognitive impairments, memory deficits, and health problems. [6-9]

Having toxic relationships or chronic stress results in anxiety, depression and even brain cell death. When your brain is exposed to an impoverished, depleted, dull environment, this neurotoxic setting produces a dull, sluggish brain. Eating poor foods leads to poor brain function. With reduced neurogenesis you don't feel well, life appears gray, threatening, sad, and hollow. With a neurotoxic lifestyle you operate below your capacity, your thinking and creativity are diminished, and problem solving ability decreases.

When neurogenesis slackens, your life slows down and deadens. Your world becomes smaller, more fixed and routine, as you move in narrow, repetitive grooves without the freshness that neurogenesis brings.

Over and over again in study after study, depression, dementia, lowered immunity, memory loss, anxiety and stress, heart disease, cancer, autoimmune diseases, loss of vitality and enjoyment, and loss of meaning are correlated with reduced neurogenesis. The evidence is clear: lowered neurogenesis means a degraded quality of life.

Neurogenesis Is the Key to the Good Life

This book is about stimulating and enhancing neurogenesis so that our brain is like an ever-renewing spring, bubbling with vitality. **A neurohealthy lifestyle brings a fulfilling life.** It creates energy, health, as well as an emotional connection to others and our own deepest center. *We are vital, alive, and engaged with life.*

A neurotoxic lifestyle, on the other hand, sends the brain into rapid decline. When the brain is exposed to toxins—whether these toxins are pollutants, stressful relationships, impoverished environments, financial strains, or lack of nutrition—the brain tries to avoid them and shuts down to protect itself from further noxious exposure. The brain's contraction, reduced neurogenesis, depression, and immobility are natural defensive reactions to poison. Everything seems ancient, decaying, mechanized as the old neural grooves repeat themselves in a spiral of entropy leading toward depression and death.

Of course, we don't consciously drink poison. Why would we deliberately choose to poison our brains? We don't. We simply get caught up in the neurotoxic patterns of the world around us and damage our brains and health unknowingly.

This is a guidebook to show the way out of neurotoxic patterns and toward neurohealthy ways of living. But some parts of this map are not simple. At times it will take thought and reflection to understand how insidious and intertwined with healthy strands some of these neurotoxic patterns are. But as we proceed, the way becomes easier to see and follow.

A neurohealthy perspective illuminates the path forward. It provides balance and a way to evaluate new situations. It allows the brain to come into its own greatest potential for clarity, openness, creativity, love, and authentic intimacy, a deep and fulfilling engagement with life in which it realizes its own deepest potential.

A Unique Moment in History

Only now, at this moment in time, with the development and convergence of several scientific disciplines, can we say with some certainty and precision what is healthy and neurogenic (stimulates neurogenesis). Conversely, we also can identify what is unhealthy and neurotoxic.

The convergence of recent findings in neuroscience, nutrition research, exercise science, depth psychology and infant research, cognitive science, interpersonal neurobiology, biochemistry, spiritual disciplines, and brain imaging reveals a map of optimal brain functioning. **This map is revolutionary, both for the individual and for society as a whole.**

No doubt, as science advances, these findings will be refined and recalibrated. Health is a moving target as scientific knowledge continually progresses. But we know so much already that it is important to act on this now. **The longer we wait, the worse things will get for us, both individually and as a species.**

The sooner we move toward a neurohealthy lifestyle, the healthier we'll be, the more joy, vitality, and love we'll generate, and the sooner our world will step back from its neurotoxic course and move toward the light of greater connection and health.

What constitutes a well-rounded brain and balanced lifestyle is unique for everyone. There is no one pattern or rigid formula. Each brain is unique and expresses an extraordinarily complex individuality. If our fingerprints are unique, our brains are infinitely more so. **You are not a type but a uniqueness.**

Neuroscience Is Too Important to Be Left to Neuroscientists

As a psychology professor for over 30 years, I've long believed that psychology is much too important to be left to psychologists. It needs to be shared with everyone. It's the same with neuroscience.

The recent discoveries of neuroscience need to be available to everyone, not buried in technical journals read only by other neuroscientists working in the same area. The possibilities for enhancing neural health are simply staggering. **Yet very little of this information gets out to the popular media, less still to the public.**

This is the problem with increasing specialization: specialists talk to other specialists in their field. Knowledge stays confined to scientific journals rather than reaching the general population. **This fragmentation of knowledge is both a blessing, in that it allows for more detailed understanding, and a curse, as the larger whole can too easily be lost.**

I'm a professor of psychology and a clinical psychologist. I teach neuroscience at the graduate level, and though I'm not a neuroscience researcher, I've watched with fascination how the field has developed in recent decades. There have been countless advances, discoveries, and an unprecedented sharing of findings between neuroscientists around the globe. Unfortunately much of the science about neurogenesis is lost to the general public, buried in esoteric PubMed abstracts. (PubMed is the U.S. Library of Medicine database for medical and life science citations.) The revolutionary implications of neurogenesis convinced me that these findings need to be known by a larger audience.

The Myth of the "Silver Bullet" for Brain Health

We all hope for a simple solution—take this pill or eat this new food—and most self-help books offer relatively easy ways to change your life for the better. But this is not your typical self-help book. When it comes to the brain, almost nothing is simple.

Given the brain's staggering complexity, a simple plan for brain health does not and cannot exist. It requires a multi-faceted approach. We need to use our whole brain to enhance our whole brain.

Brain health is key to health in every area—physical, emotional, mental, spiritual. As present trends continue, 50% of adults aged 85 or older can expect to receive a diagnosis of Alzheimer's disease, which is marked by a dramatic loss of brain cells, especially in the hippocampus. Since most of the adult population today is expected to live longer than 85, this means you have about a 50-50 chance of developing Alzheimer's. What's the point of keeping the body alive longer if you lose your mind?

Getting older doesn't have to be a downward spiral. Aging can mean getting wiser, deeper, more creative, more interesting and more interested, more joyful, more peaceful, more awake to the present moment, and evolving into a more loving human being. **But for this to occur, you need to renew and enhance your brain's capacities, and this brings us to neurogenesis.**

Without a change in values and lifestyle, modern culture will become even more neurotoxic and consequently there will be marked increases in stress, depression, illness due to lowered immunity, obesity, diabetes, Alzheimer's and dementia, ADD/ADHD, autism, and other forms of brain dysfunction. But that's all avoidable if you know what to do. **Consider this book your guide to healthy aging.**

Your brain wants you to use it, otherwise you lose it. Using it means engaging your brain on all levels through your lifestyle.

Future Dreams

In the future, our understanding of neurogenesis will hopefully develop to the point that neurodegenerative diseases and crippling spinal cord injuries will be not only be treatable but curable. In the "bad old days" of the early decades of the 21st century there is no way to regenerate lost brain tissue, but as neurogenesis becomes better understood it will be possible to not only stop the rapid death of brain cells in Alzheimer's disease sufferers but to grow new neurons so the person is able to regain lost cognitive functions.

With Parkinson's disease, stopping the loss of dopamine neurons will be followed by a careful targeted stimulation of neurogenesis which guides new neuron development into dopamine neurons to replace those that were lost so normal movement is restored.

In the future, other neurodegenerative diseases, such as multiple sclerosis (MS), ALS (Lou Gehrig's disease), Huntington's, and other types of dementia, will be routinely cured as neurogenesis becomes more fully understood.

Spinal cord injuries that now sentence a person to life as a paraplegic or quadriplegic will be just temporary, treatable conditions. With targeted neurogenesis, the neurons along the spine can regrow across the severed connections. Wheelchairs will be a rarity in the future, used only as a short-term transition until full movement is regained. In short, the possibilities improved neurogenesis research brings are nearly limitless and their practical applications have the potential to change the world. Only time will tell.

Summary

In the past decade, neuroscience has discovered that your brain is capable of performing at a much, much higher level, even in your "prime" years. We don't yet know the upper limits of our potentials. Yet as momentous as these discoveries are, they are practically unknown.

We do know the key is neurogenesis, which is the birth of new brain cells. The rate of neurogenesis is an indicator of how well you're functioning, cognitively, emotionally, and physically. Neurogenesis happens throughout your entire life, though it normally slows in middle age and even more in old age. However, it's now been discovered that your rate of neurogenesis can increase dramatically in all stages of adulthood, changing the entire quality of your life.

This book is for adults of all ages. Your brain can renew itself at any time. **But the earlier you begin the proper care and feeding of your brain, the greater the results.** Beginning in your twenties, thirties, or forties will achieve more powerful results than starting in your seventies or eighties, but a great deal can be done whenever you start.

You can upgrade your brain. You can operate at a higher level than ever before thought possible. This book shows you how.

CHAPTER 2

THE PROGRAM:

ENHANCE YOUR WHOLE BRAIN

If you are to become all that you can be, the health of your brain is of the highest importance. **To realize your greatest potential requires your brain to operate at its peak level.** Anything that interferes with your brain function degrades your whole quality of life. Conversely, whatever helps your brain to function at a higher level will help fulfill your potential.

A vibrant brain with a high rate of neurogenesis is the goal.

Everyone wants their brain to be healthy, to function at its highest capacity. But there is so much that is neurotoxic in our environment that no one escapes unscathed. Life throws a lot of obstacles our way, which we then internalize as bad habits and inflict upon ourselves.

Throughout our lives we all suffer hurts and injuries of various kinds—physical, emotional, mental, spiritual. Even "normal aging" has so much unnecessary toxicity that the brain declines much faster than it needs to. But this is far from inevitable.

You can design a lifestyle that promotes neurogenesis and avoids the main neurotoxic assaults of daily life. It's a two-fold strategy: increase what's neurohealthy and decrease what's neurotoxic.

A Holistic Plan to Enhance Neurogenesis

The brain wants to engage with life and people through the senses and emotion, through mental stimulation and in spiritual freedom. The brain is an extraordinary instrument honed by millions of years of evolution. Its vast complexity cannot be reduced to mapping synapses or fiddling with a few neurotransmitters. Only a holistic understanding of the brain can do justice to its complex wholeness.

I confess a part of me wishes I could just take a pill to increase my rate of neurogenesis. It would make it all so simple. **But the thing about the brain is that nothing is simple.** I've learned to be suspicious of quick fixes when it comes to brain health.

If the research shows anything, it is that there is no magic pill to enhance neurogenesis. If anyone offers you such a wondrous drug, run screaming in the other direction, for this is at best a hoax and at worst a pact with the devil (and we all know how that will turn out). But while the path to brain health is neither quick nor easy, it is accessible to nearly everyone. Everything you need to increase neurogenesis is available right now, and most of it for free.

The New Holism

Holism understands we are complex beings that cannot be reduced to separate parts. The human organism operates as an integrated whole and can only be understood in the context of this wholeness. If a person loses a leg, it changes how the entire organism balances and moves. If hearing is lost, the other senses increase to compensate. When someone is angry, it is expressed on physical, emotional, mental, and spiritual levels. Anything we do, think, see, or feel is experienced as an interrelated whole.

Originally inspired by 20th century Indian sage Sri Aurobindo's integral philosophy, the new holism corrects and expands the partial European view of holism put forward in the early 1920s and popularized in the 1960s. The first holism was a product of the European Enlightenment and so focused only on the empirical unity of body-heart-mind. When this original holistic paradigm first came on the American scene in the 1960s it was a welcome advance over the reductionist thinking prevalent at that time. **However, it was incomplete in that it left out our most essential element: spirit.**

Sri Aurobindo, considered by many as the greatest Vedantic philosopher of all time, corrected this oversight by incorporating spirit as the foundation of human consciousness. If the level of spirit is not included, our picture is incomplete. We miss the defining element of being human. **Body, heart, and mind are the outer instruments for an evolving soul or spirit.** But only by including all four levels of our being is the human formula complete: body, heart, mind, spirit.

Holism 2.0: Body, Heart, Mind, Spirit

The only way to fully understand the brain is through a broad view that encompasses all of its possibilities for consciousness. Each level of body, heart, mind, and spirit has its own vibration or energy frequency, with the physical body being the densest and therefore having the lowest frequency.

Every level—physical, emotional, mental, spiritual—has its own "consciousness" that is experienced through the brain and contributes to the whole that is you. Only by considering all four levels can the brain be fully understood and thus allowed its highest development.

Purely physical or material approaches that try to understand the brain from the bottom up are woefully inadequate and leave out much that is essential. The majority of conventional neuroscience literature reduces the miracle of the human being to a cluster of neurotransmitters or biological processes divorced from relationships, beauty, and spirit.

In researching this book I was continually struck by the small, drab worldview that many (but not all) neuroscience researchers put forth. The picture of the brain that emerges from a purely materialistic worldview is a shrunken, pale reflection of the brain's magnificence. It is sadly reductionistic, like trying to squeeze the glory and immensity of human consciousness into a laboratory beaker. Such a partial, one-dimensional focus is no doubt helpful at times but only as a temporary measure, and it is to the integrated wholeness of the brain that we must always return.

We exist and live on different levels simultaneously. Each level of who we are—body, heart, mind, spirit—finds expression through the brain. Honoring our whole brain means bringing forth the unique ways our whole body-heart-mind-spirit expresses itself in the world.

It's All In Your Head

Remember, everything we experience, we experience through the brain. A holistic approach to brain health opens up all four levels of our being, for the brain supports them all.

- **Body:** The body is your foundation. Sensing the world and moving within it grounds you in your physical being—from the passing clouds to the smile on a child's face, from the simple sensory pleasure of water on your skin in the shower to the joy of walking or exercising, from the sound of music to the delight of eating a tasty meal. When the senses and body are stimulated, so is this level of the brain.
- **Heart:** The heart signifies your emotional level. You are alive to the extent that you can feel. When you diminish your feelings, you diminish your aliveness. Expanding your capacity for intimacy, love, and connection is one of life's most precious gifts and stimulates neurogenesis, for the brain is wired for emotional relationships. With negative relationships and chronic feelings of stress and depression this capacity shrinks—and so does neurogenesis. When we live in mostly positive emotional states, with safety and love, our emotional brains expand and so, accordingly, does neurogenesis.
- **Mind:** Your ability to learn throughout your lifespan makes life endlessly fascinating. Learning is not restricted to memorizing facts in school but includes learning about

the whole of life, right hemisphere as well as left. The joy of mental stimulation, whether through story-telling, conversing, reading, thinking, enjoying music, or fantasizing, stretches and stimulates the mind and neurogenesis.

- **Spirit:** Spirituality is the highest value in most people's lives and the guiding light of almost every culture throughout history. Spiritual practices work to purify our dense outer natures and reveal our deeper souls or spirits. Awakening to our deeper spiritual beings through practices such as mindfulness and heart opening, aspiration techniques, prayer, and compassion have profound effects upon the brain's renewal and growth.

A reductionistic, purely physical view of the brain leads to one-sided development and ignores what is most essential to our human brains. **Whole brain health means engaging all four levels of our being.** While enhancing neurogenesis on one level is certainly better than nothing, optimally we want to enhance our whole brain along all four dimensions. Giving free play to our brain's extraordinary capacities at every stage of life means keeping neurogenesis high through a lifestyle that supports it.

This is a holistic plan to enhance our whole brain, for only by including body, heart, mind, and spirit can we fully appreciate the magnificence of our brains' possibilities and stimulate all dimensions of neurogenesis.

A Cafeteria-Style Plan

This book spells out a plan to safely increase neurogenesis by stimulating all levels of the brain (body, heart, mind, and spirit) while simultaneously reducing exposure to neurotoxins that slow it down. It is divided into chapters that address each level.

I'd suggest a quick read-through of the whole book first, and then come back to the key sections you most want to focus on. Don't worry about taking on everything at once. The amount of information here can seem overwhelming if you try to tackle it all in one go. Instead, start with the sections that most appeal to you and then add the rest in time.

Since diet is such a key part of brain health, an entire chapter is devoted to it. There are some foods that increase neurogenesis and support brain health and are therefore helpful to include in your diet. There are other foods that it would be wise to avoid or minimize as they decrease neurogenesis. But diet isn't everything. There are other physical things to do, which is the focus of the chapter after diet.

Additionally, there are emotional ways of engaging the world that are important for neurogenesis and neural health. There are mental forms of stimulation that are neurogenic. And there are spiritual practices to include for well-rounded neural development.

Equally important is not slowing down neurogenesis by engaging in activities that reduce the process of forming new brain cells. A later chapter focuses on things to avoid or minimize in order to enhance neurogenesis so you don't undermine your progress toward higher levels of well-being. The final chapter puts it all together.

Leaving out any one level reduces what you can achieve, so include body, heart, mind, and spirit, but within each level pick and choose those practices that best fit you.

At first, focus on what you're most drawn to. Design your own unique path to brain enhancement. Do what's right for you now and trust this will take you where you need to go. The rest will come in its own time as you're ready.

Think of the various ways to increase neurogenesis as items in a cafeteria. Pick and choose what you want. Some things will seem right immediately, others will seem foreign or unappealing. **Experiment. Try out different approaches.** Don't feel compelled to do everything right away, rather find your own path. Do what feels right, and let the rest go for now. Simply try to pick methods from each level: body, heart, mind, and spirit.

Each of us must take responsibility for the health of our own brain. How much or how little we do is up to us alone. It's not even possible to do everything, to take every substance or participate in every neurogenic activity. Some of this is trial and error. Accept that you have limits like every human being while knowing it's possible to increase your rate of neurogenesis and operate at a higher level in daily life.

Recent research shows that some methods for increasing neurogenesis only work along certain parts of the hippocampus. This is why an inclusive strategy for increasing neurogenesis is needed to stimulate the entire hippocampus—one that incorporates all four levels, not just the body. Otherwise only certain areas of the brain may thrive while other areas wither away.

The Central Secret

If this becomes work, something is wrong. The brain is wired for pleasure, for joy, for love, for interest and excitement, for meaning and depth, for passion and creativity, for learning and wonder. If there is pain in this, it only comes as we withdraw from some of our toxic addictions. But this temporary discomfort has a speedy recompense in the form of greater health, healing, wholeness, joy, love, and flow as our brains quickly adapt to a higher level of functioning.

A holistic approach to developing the brain means engaging with life in all its dimensions—physical, emotional, mental, spiritual. Our personal growth and our brains' growth are one.

When we grow we feel good, like we've come into ourselves more fully. **We have only one thing to do in this life: to become our best self.** There is no one pattern or type that we should try to emulate, rather we should simply become ourselves, individuating into our own uniqueness at every level.

This is a map for that journey.

The Brain Determines *Everything* in Your Life

Ponder this for a moment: everything you experience, you experience through the brain. There is nothing you see, hear, feel, or think that doesn't come to you through your brain. Every moment of your life, every hope, every memory, every love or hate, triumph or defeat, every sight and smell and taste—**every single thing comes to you through your brain.**

When you really understand how critical your brain is to *everything* you do, you will naturally want your brain to be the healthiest and best it can be.

Most people know the human brain is the most complex thing in the known universe but don't appreciate the scale of this complexity. Consider these facts:

1. The neuron (brain cell) is the most complicated cell in the human body. Neurons have primary dendrites that branch out like the roots of a tree into secondary and tertiary

dendrites and connect to other neurons via synapses. On each of these branches are thousands of synaptic connections with other neurons. Some neurons have over a thousand branching dendrites that connect them to tens of thousands of other neurons. Most neurons fire impulses at a rate of about 10–100 times per second, depending upon the type of neuron.

2. The adult brain has an estimated 100 billion brain cells.
3. Each neuron is connected to an average of 7,000–10,000 other neurons, some far more. Most adults have around 100 trillion synapses.

Such vast interconnection presents us with a breathtaking degree of complexity. Like the number of stars in the sky, these numbers are too large to comprehend. Further, the brain operates with multiple redundancies, complex protective mechanisms, backup systems, and alternate pathways of communication that maintain a homeostatic balance we are only beginning to understand. In its 600 million year evolution the brain has developed numerous ways to correct imbalances and protect itself against outside assaults.

There are about 50 known neurotransmitters, and may be many more, each can have up to 14 different kinds of receptors that recognize them. How these neurotransmitters "converse" with each other through multi-layered feedback systems presents a staggering array of possibilities for complex interactions. Over 20 neurotransmitters, for example, are involved in emotion and mood regulation, as well as many of the over 80 known hormones. **The communication *among and between* different neurotransmitters, hormones, and neuromodulators adds new layers of complexity**

to already unfathomable complexity. Our understanding of the brain's complexity hardly amounts to a scratch on the surface.

For a more complete overview of the brain, please read **Appendix A: A Brief Tour of Your Brain** at the back of this book.

Humility

It seems advisable to me to approach studying the extraordinary wonder that is the human brain with an attitude of great humility and to be prepared to drop a favored theory in an instant when the science shows disconfirming data. Although many in the neuroscience community share this sense of wonder and humility, unfortunately many others do not.

Neuroscience, like any infant science, can occasionally be brash, arrogant, and make assertions that go well beyond the data. At times it seems like most any theory *du jour* can find justification through a neuroscience explanation.

Similarly, the hubris and simplistic thinking that accompany changing the brain's chemistry by increasing or decreasing one neurotransmitter or another is a bit like handing a five-year-old a scalpel and expecting him to do brain surgery. The child is so far out of his depth he has no idea of the damage he can wreak. Even though medication can sometimes help, such powerful drugs often have major unintended consequences.

It is very tempting to believe in simple solutions to problems involving the extraordinary complexity of the brain. **But because of its many protective systems, the brain cannot be manipulated like a chemical in a test tube.** It reacts to such intrusions on many levels by increasing or decreasing other chemicals and neurotransmitters in its infinitely complex electro-chemical conversation, a dialogue that goes far beyond our current ability to even track, let alone understand, what is going on. This leaves aside the unknown number of peptides, hormones, and neurotransmitters that have not yet even been discovered.

The Question of Evidence

Scientific understanding of what is going on in the human brain is often based on study and analysis of mammals who have similar brains to humans. Even with increased brain imaging techniques, which are growing more powerful daily, most of what we know about the human brain we've learned from mammal brains, since experiments with human brains are necessarily much more limited. Researchers can't kill a human being after an experiment to examine his or her brain like they can with a mouse. **However, humans share common mechanisms with other mammalian brains,** which is why mammals are used in research.

Mammal brains have the same basic structures. Almost all experiments have shown matching effects in mammals and humans. **All mammals have brains built with the same architecture.** The mouse brain, monkey brain, and human brain differ in the amount and complexity of their systems, but the basic structures are identical. For example, the neurocortex of humans is 30% of the brain, whereas in monkeys it is only 12% and 3% in cats. But the basic structures remain the same across species.

Human, mouse, monkey, and other mammal brains share the same neurotransmitters as well as the same brain structures. Antidepressant drugs such as SSRIs, SNRIs, and NDRIs work in the same way across mammalian species. Stress and depression have similar effects in humans, mice, and monkeys.

As in all areas of science there are some controversies over what certain data mean. For example, mice, monkeys, and humans all share a limbic system, or emotional brain. While such states as stress or depression look physiologically and behaviorally identical in all three species, some researchers describe stressful or depressive-like behavior in mice and monkeys rather than say they feel stressed or depressed—after all, animals can't articulate their emotions. Interestingly, many of the researchers who actually work with mice or monkeys believe that they do indeed *feel* stress and depression and so use these terms in their articles.

After neurogenesis was discovered in other mammals, it took almost two decades to show definitively that neurogenesis also occurs in adult humans. Many researchers resisted the idea of neurogenesis in humans since it conflicted with the long-held belief that no new brain cells formed after adulthood. **But once that cherished myth was dispelled and the new paradigm of adult neurogenesis was ushered in, many researchers wondered why it had taken so long to generalize brain findings from mammals to humans.**

There is no current way to directly measure the rate of neurogenesis in humans, aside from brain dissection after death. Neuroimaging studies that show increased blood flow or increased brain volume in specific areas are highly suggestive of neurogenesis but not definitive the way a postmortem autopsy is.

However, since humans live much longer than other mammals, it can take decades before subjects die and their brains can be properly examined.

Do you want to wait for decades of further cognitive decline to be certain that, for example, a particular nutrient that stimulates neurogenesis in other mammals also works in humans? Or would you rather know now what the research shows and make your own choices about what to use in your own life? If the latter, then continue reading.

Many of the findings of neuroscience, as in all science, are subject to interpretation. Some neuroscience interpretations are more conservative while others take the same set of facts and run wild with them, such as many brain-training games that research says are mostly worthless but are still wildly promoted under the guise of neuroscience. This book attempts to stick closely to what the research has revealed and adopts a middle of the road approach to interpreting these data—which will no doubt draw disagreements from both sides. There are times when the data are suggestive but not yet definitive, and in these cases this is clearly identified so the reader can make an informed judgment.

In some areas science moves forward at breakneck speed. In other areas it progresses at a pace that is agonizingly slow. Miraculous breakthroughs move the field forward in leaps and bounds, yet confirming studies can take years or even decades.

The best data we have now indicates that the neurogenic effects of practices put forward in this book occur across species, but only further research will make these assumptions absolutely definitive. As with any book about science, there will no doubt be some modifications as research moves forward, for science is always a moving target. However, I imagine the vast majority of the information in this book will be confirmed as studies continue.

It's worth noting that most neuroscientists who study neurogenesis are using many of these same practices in their own lives. In speaking about the strong increase in neurogenesis from running wheels in mice, Fred Gage, Ph.D., was asked by the interviewer about his own practices. He replied that yes, this discovery led him to run in his own life and most other neuroscience researchers he knew also exercised. [1] It is this sort of information that is offered in this book.

Heraclitus's Brain

Physics describes a universe of continual flux and change. The Greek philosopher Heraclitus captured this flowing nature of existence with his maxim, "You never step into the same river twice." The same can be said for the brain. **You never experience the same brain twice.**

It's a mistake to think of the brain as a solid "thing" like a computer. Its composition is more like a soufflé that hasn't fully set or soft Jell-O. In many ways the brain is closer to a slow moving fluid than stable matter. It's sheltered by the bony skull, encased in layers of soft tissue, and suspended in protective cerebrospinal fluid.

The brain is extremely delicate. Remember, the so-called wiring is not like a metal wire at all. No neurons actually touch each other; instead there's a space between neurons, a synapse across which they communicate using electro-chemical signals. After a signal is sent, the chemical messenger is absorbed again so the synapse is cleared and ready to send another signal.

The brain's breathtaking complexity exists in a highly sensitive, fragile environment, which is why a head injury or sharp jolt can damage this "wiring" and disrupt the delicate synaptic connections.

The brain is in a constant state of change and flux, always adapting to new input, transforming with every sound, every sight, every sensation, thought, feeling, image, and desire. Within minutes of being in a new environment, your brain has changed considerably to adapt to it. Reading this sentence is changing your brain right now.

Everything we experience changes the brain. It has to. Each thing we see, each sound we hear registers as some kind of alteration in the brain. If the brain isn't altered by input, there is no experience. Think of the brain as a giant amoeba, ever moving, ever adapting, ever sensing its environment and responding.

As the brain changes and adapts, it constantly creates new connections among brain cells. With repetition, these changes rewire the brain. As early neuropsychology researcher Donald Hebb famously said, **"Neurons that fire together wire together."** Over time this creates neural pathways and neural networks that make routine tasks easy and habitual.

Without repetition, however, most neural connections are pruned and disappear. Indeed, the brain is highly efficient at eliminating unused connections. This makes sense given the limited space of the skull. There's only room for the essentials.

The brain is continually modeling and remodeling itself. Up until recently it was believed that brain plasticity was very limited and became even more limited with age. Since brain cells only died and were never replaced, it was mistakenly thought, the best we could hope for was new connections among existing brain cells achieved by learning new things.

New research has upended this dreary picture of aging. Not only are new brain cells created from neuronal stem cells but brain plasticity is a dynamic source of renewal. Indeed, the brain can recover from injury and trauma much more fully than previously believed, especially when brain healthy principles are followed. The living brain is in constant flux.

Movement Is Life, Stasis Is Death

An optimally stimulated, flowing brain has high neurogenesis and neural plasticity. It is dynamic. In contrast, a depressed brain is sluggish and slow moving. It has very reduced neurogenesis. Plasticity too is reduced, compromised, inhibited. It's almost as if depression does to the brain *physically* what it does to the person *emotionally*—it slows things down. It even shrinks the brain. Depressed people have a smaller hippocampus than non-depressed people. The more depressive episodes, the greater the brain shrinkage, possibly due to more episodes of reduced neurogenesis. Death occurs when movement stops altogether.

Looking at adult brains more carefully has shown that the number of adult neurons is fairly stable and durable. Studies that count the number of cells show little or no difference in the number of brain cells in older people. This picture changes, however, with disease. Alzheimer's disease, Parkinson's, and myriad other diseases dramatically kill off neurons. Depression, alcohol use, chronic stress or acute and intense stress, inflammation, and other toxins also reduce brain size and slow neurogenesis.

The Goldilocks Problem in Brain Growth

When you live in a small apartment, you need to make everything count. You need the essentials, but if too much junk piles up you're drowned in clutter. What you bring in needs to be balanced by what you throw out. This is similar to the problem faced by the brain in its evolutionary development.

Think for a moment about the problem nature confronted when dealing with the twin problems of **how to protect the delicate, sensitive tissue of the brain while at the same time allowing for new growth.** On the one hand, encasing the delicate brain protects it from injury. But this same protective casing limits how big it can grow. If the brain grows too big it will damage other brain cells by smashing them against the enclosed space in the skull, and the organism will die out in the evolutionary struggle. It's a Goldilocks problem: the balance between pruning old neurons and growing new ones needs to be just right.

The hippocampus solves this problem with staggering precision. The brain continually prunes new neurons and connections that are not used, which is essential to avoid over clutter. The brain is composed mainly of neurons and glial cells, which help hold neurons in place as well as protecting, cleaning, and pruning the brain. Glial cells are continuously on the lookout for synapses and neurons that aren't being used so they can eliminate them.

At the same time, to cope with an ever-evolving environment, new brain growth needs to focus on the most essential new elements of the inner and outer world. **The hippocampus performs this task perfectly.**

Why the Hippocampus Is So Important for Neurogenesis

Although there have been reports of neurogenesis in other areas of the brain, the only areas where it is confirmed to occur are the olfactory bulb that processes smells and the hippocampus. The hippocampus has been extensively studied by now. **What is so remarkable about the hippocampus is that it is central to all four levels of our humanness, namely:** *body, heart, mind, and spirit.*

New neurons produced by the hippocampus take about three or four weeks to mature. They then migrate to an area of the hippocampus where they are needed and integrate into the existing circuitry. These new neurons soon become identical to older, sister neurons that have existed for decades. So rather than growing neurons willy-nilly, the hippocampus produces new neurons that then respond to the stimulation that evokes them—physical, emotional, mental, spiritual. The hippocampus is involved in:

- physical movement, exercise, and spatial learning (body)
- mood and emotion, especially stress, anxiety, fear, and depression (heart)
- cognition, learning, and new memory formation (mind)
- spiritual practices such as mindfulness, devotion, and compassion (spirit)

The hippocampus is a master key that is centrally involved in all dimensions of human consciousness. It is the ideal location to produce new brain cells that keep the brain self-renewing.

The hippocampus is a curved structure that looks like a crescent moon or a curled silkworm. The hippocampus has two ends, the temporal (or ventral) and the septal (or dorsal).

The septal end is most involved in memory, new learning, and cognition. This side connects to other brain systems that mediate body awareness and spatial processing as well as thinking and learning (body and mind). The hippocampus doesn't store new memories, rather it *processes* them, aggregates their different features (sensory-emotional-cognitive meanings) and organizes them into coherent memories that give us a feeling of continuity in time and space.

The temporal end, on the other hand, is more involved in regulating emotion, especially stress and depression (in other words, the often-overlooked level of the heart). This end connects to other brain systems in the limbic system that process emotion, including the amygdala. **When neurogenesis is high in this portion of the hippocampus a person (or mouse or monkey) has strong emotional resources to deal with stress, fear, anxiety, loneliness, and depression-inducing events.**[13]

However, as we'll learn more about when examining the neurotoxic effects of stress, strong and chronic (over months or years) stress can actually kill neurons in the hippocampus. This leaves the person (or mouse or monkey) much more vulnerable to future stress and anxiety and creates one kind of PTSD (post-traumatic stress disorder).[12]

The overall size of the entire hippocampus is impacted by spiritual practices such as meditation (the level of spirit). With spiritual practice the entire length of the hippocampus enlarges.

If we had to pick one part of the brain that would keep us young and alive, we'd want to pick the part that was key to our whole functioning. In other words, we'd pick the hippocampus.

Further, since particular kinds of stimulation produce new neurons that are specific to that stimulation, **having a wide variety of strategies for neurogenesis will result in the widest, most complete renewal of the whole brain.** One-sided strategies bring partial results. A holistic approach to brain health is the most inclusive and effective strategy possible.

Will This Program Work?

I not only believe this is the most effective way to upgrade your brain and life, it is a program I use myself. It's the most comprehensive understanding of what constitutes an enriched environment, and there are several lines of evidence to support this holistic approach. First, the research data shows that providing an enriched environment stimulates the brain in multiple ways with a synergetic effect. That is, separate kinds of neurogenic activity—such as exercise, diet, emotional, and cognitive stimulation—work together more powerfully than they do apart.

Different kinds of brain stimulation support each other. For instance, running boosts neurogenesis but with running alone there is a 40–60% loss of these newly created brain cells. However, other parts of an enriched environment prevent neuronal cell loss but don't increase the number of new neurons formed. Put together there is a large boost in new brain cells as well as an almost 100% survival rate. But only a holistic, multi-pronged approach produces the powerful boost in both new neurons and survival rates that results in a major increase in neurogenesis.

A second line of research evidence comes from one research center with a larger vision. Currently, research in the Americas and Europe is overwhelmingly driven by financial concerns—pharmaceutical companies fund much of the research. Researchers looking to find the next big (selling) drug do much of the rest; for example it is possible to slightly tweak the molecular structure of a natural compound that has some biological effect so that this tweaked version can then be patented—regardless of its efficacy. The lure of money distorts the research agenda to an appalling degree.

There are a few research centers, however, that are beginning to look at the bigger picture. One of these is the Buck Institute for Research on Aging in Novato, California. Shortly before this book went to press, in the October 2014 issue of the journal *Aging*, researchers from the Buck Institute and UCLA reported the first known success for reversing Alzheimer's disease. **Researchers using a simplified version of the strategy outlined in this book found greater success than had ever before been achieved.**

Thus far the prevailing wisdom insisted that by the time Alzheimer's is noticed or diagnosed, there is so much damage to the brain that it's irreversible and unstoppable. Like someone falling down a cliff, nature must take its course and the descent into increasing neural devastation is inevitable.

Indeed, billions have been invested to find a chemical compound that will stop or reverse the mental decline of Alzheimer's—with no success. Hundreds of clinical trials costing many billions of dollars have taken place, resulting only in failure after failure to even slow the disease's progression. Drugs have only had modest, temporary effects on symptoms. Nothing seemed to work.

Using a simplified version of this book's system, a pilot study found that memory loss may be reversed and the improvement sustained with this program. The study involved changing diet along some of the guidelines discussed in this book (such as eliminating sugar, reducing carbohydrates and processed food, and adding more vegetables and non-farmed salmon), plus adding just a few of the supplements included in the "Diet" chapter, in conjunction with exercise, better sleep, and meditation.

Nine of the ten patients had a strong positive response to this program. Those who had left work due to memory problems or who were struggling at work were able to return to their employment with improved performance. These improvements have been sustained for two and a half years and counting after initial treatment.

Although this study was aimed at helping Alzheimer's patients, it included things that also happen to stimulate neurogenesis. Hopefully this study is just the first step toward proving greater brain health can be achieved using the holistic strategy laid out here. In contrast, this book focuses primarily upon increasing neurogenesis, with neurohealthy aging and Alzheimer's prevention as additional benefits.

A third line of data comes from clinical experience. My clinical practice with clients shows strong support for this approach. Using a neurogenesis-informed treatment strategy, I find my clients respond extremely well after just a few months. However, I have observed it takes a good year or two of following this program to create the most robust, rock solid foundation in brain function and really feel the internal boost. **Clients report feeling better than**

they've ever felt in their lives, with more energy and enthusiasm, more mental acuity and sharpness, and greater confidence than they believed possible.

"I've never felt so good in my life!" is a common remark. Such evidence is considered anecdotal, but it certainly shows where future research needs to go. The best evidence will come from your own observations when you compare your present experience to where you'll be in a year or two.

The following chapters are diligently researched and present only demonstrated methods for increasing neurogenesis and brain health.

How the Brain Grows

What stimulates neurogenesis and neural growth are various chemical messengers known as "neurotrophins." These include nerve growth factor (NGF) and neurotrophin-3 (NT-3), which are involved with sensory neurons, and other neurotrophins that are less well understood. One of the best studied is called brain-derived neurotrophic factor, or BDNF for short. It appears to be the main signal that turns on neurogenesis. Increasing neurogenesis means increasing BDNF levels as well.

An enriched environment increases BDNF levels in the brain, stimulating neurogenesis and neural growth.

Increasing BDNF levels also means decreasing your exposure to the four poisons highlighted in the chapter "Increase Neurogenesis By Not Slowing It Down." These four poisons are:

- chronic inflammation
- chronic stress (including anxiety and fear)
- physical assaults
- deprivation

Brain health depends not only on new brain cells forming but on their survival. In normal neurogenesis about 60–70% of new neurons die off. Some ways of increasing neurogenesis can lower this figure to 40–60%. However, in a highly enriched environment almost all new neurons survive. Thus, our best hope for optimal brain vitality is both to increase the rate of neurogenesis *and* to increase the survival rate for these new brain cells. **BDNF is important for both the birth and survival of newborn neurons.**

The question then becomes: how do we increase BDNF in a healthy way?

Note the last four words of that question: "in a healthy way."

Researchers learned early on that increasing levels of BDNF too much results in impaired brain and memory function. That is, artificially raising BDNF levels by injecting brain-derived neurotrophic factor directly into the brain has the opposite effect from what would be expected. Too much BDNF interferes with cognition, new memory formation, and neurogenesis. Remember, the brain is this extraordinarily complex system of checks and balances, with multiple protective mechanisms. Just manually adding extra BDNF to the brain's "soup" can seriously impair how the brain works.

Protect Your Most Precious Asset—Your Brain

We need to work *with* the brain to increase BDNF levels and *include* the brain's protective mechanisms, rather than try to bypass them. **The focus of this book is working *with* the brain to enhance neurogenesis.** There are healthy, effective ways to do this.

This book proposes safe, natural ways for increasing neurogenesis that respect the brain's defenses rather than trying to override them.

What does the brain want? It wants to engage the world and use its capacities, to fulfill its potential. It wants us to thrive, to love, to enjoy at all levels: body, heart, mind, spirit. Why wouldn't we want to align with this?

Future Dreams

In the future, after neuroimaging capabilities increase, it will become possible to measure the exact rates of neurogenesis in each part of the hippocampus. When a patient comes to see a doctor complaining of not feeling well and forgetting things, the physician will be able to test her brain and say, "Yes, the septal end of your hippocampus is only working at 50% of capacity for neurogenesis, while the temporal end is only at 35%. Of course you feel anxious, depressed, and are forgetting things."

The prescription the doctor will give the patient will show how far medicine has evolved. No longer will doctors bludgeon the brain with one or two heavy drugs and hope for the best. Instead the patient will be given a holistic range of interventions to focus on each level of body, heart, mind, and spirit that target the specific regions of the hippocampus that need stimulation.

Two months later when she comes back in, the doctor will look at the neuroimaging and say, "Excellent! It looks like you're back up to 90% in both areas of your hippocampus. How do you feel?" The patient will report feeling better, in fact so much better she's realized she wants to change careers and is going back to school. "I didn't realize how much my job stress was grinding me down. This was just the wake-up call I needed."

Summary

Partial, one-sided materialistic biases in much (but not all) of science reduce human experience to a fraction of what it is and disregards what is most essential in human life. **The full glory of the human brain, with its extraordinary range of consciousness, often gets left behind in the research lab.** Every part of us wants to grow, not just certain select parts. Seeing the brain holistically lets us understand and develop our abilities at all levels: body, heart, mind, spirit.

The brain is perhaps the ultimate Rorschach test. Whatever we bring to our study of the brain we can find, for the brain is large enough to hold it all. This book advocates that only the largest, widest, and most comprehensive view of human consciousness can do justice to the discoveries of neuroscience and the possibilities for renewal that neurogenesis offers.

When we embrace all of who we are, we allow our highest potentials to flower. To increase neurogenesis, we begin with diet, then move on to body, heart, mind, spirit, and finally conclude with things to avoid that slow it down.

CHAPTER 3

DIET

This chapter focuses on foods that promote neurogenesis and brain health. A growing body of research shows that, beyond increasing neurogenesis, a neurohealthy diet protects against stress, depression, and Alzheimer's. This chapter is organized into three sections:

- First, there are numerous foods, nutrients, spices, and plant extracts that increase neurogenesis.
- Second, there are dozens more that increase BDNF levels and *may* also increase neurogenesis, but the confirming data aren't in yet.
- The third section describes principles of a neurohealthy diet that supports neurogenesis and optimizes brain function. This diet protects the brain from inflammation, oxidation, and glycation. It also details the foods that slow neurogenesis, damage brain health, and are better minimized or avoided altogether.

At the end of the chapter are charts that summarize this.

Mary

Mary first came to see me complaining of high levels of stress at her work, combined with bouts of depression and fears about her declining memory. In her late thirties, she was the head attorney for an iconic Fortune 500 company. She was showing signs of metabolic syndrome: higher glucose levels, increasing belly fat weight gain, higher blood pressure, loss of libido. Her wicked sense of humor endeared her to her co-workers, and though she was highly competent, she had real insecurities about herself and her job performance. She worked the corporate legal field like a pro but never felt that she was doing enough.

A holistic assessment revealed the roots of her complaints in each level of body, heart, mind, and spirit.

We did some work around her beliefs and spiritual life, but a cold and emotionally distant mother was at the center of her fragile sense of self-esteem. This early relationship made all relationships feel dangerous, so she kept people at arm's length. As a way to feel love and a sense of safety, she'd turned to eating comfort foods. She was a good example of the all-American diet: high sugar, high carb, fast and fried foods were her staples.

While healing her early wounds through our therapeutic relationship and connecting with her young, vulnerable self was important, she made dramatic shifts in her mood by changing her diet. The very foods she ate to feel comforted and soothed were the very foods that made her susceptible to stress and depression, they even interfered with memory as well as inhibited neurogenesis.

"The first two weeks of cutting down on sugar, chocolate, and pasta were the hardest," she later said. "But then when I was able to eat plenty of healthy, high fat foods that I used to avoid like the plague, this took the edge off and made me feel calmer, more solid in myself."

After six months much of her belly fat melted away, but it was the mood change that most surprised her. Adding fish oil, green tea, turmeric, and blueberries to her new low sugar diet clearly had a big effect on her rate of neurogenesis. "My job stress barely seems like a big deal now, and depressive thoughts hardly even come anymore," she shared one day. "I never would've believed that what I eat has such a big impact on how I feel."

Foods and Nutrients that Stimulate Neurogenesis

All of the foods and nutrients below are available as extracts. This makes including these in your diet more economical and practical. For example, a daily diet that includes fresh blueberries can be pricey, but two capsules of blueberry extract is much more affordable and easier to keep in the house. The following nutrients have been shown to increase neurogenesis:

- blueberries
- omega-3 fatty acids, (especially DHA and EPA) extracts from fish oil (or flax oil or algae)
- green tea and green tea extracts containing the catechin EGCG
- curcumin, from the spice turmeric (found in curry)
- whole soy foods such as tofu, edamame, soy milk, soy nuts, and soy isoflavone extracts containing daidzein and genistein
- ginseng extract
- ginkgo biloba (an herbal extract)
- quercetin (found in many foods and sold as an extract)

- vitamin E
- piperine (found in pepper)
- DHEA and pregnenolone
- tryptophan and 5-HTP
- rhodiola, aka rose root
- melatonin
- mulberry
- red sage, aka danshen and salvia
- lithium
- goji Berry, aka wolfberry
- grape seed extract
- lotus root extract
- apigenin
- luteolin

Many of these foods and nutrients may be taken daily or several times a week. With some of them, taking the right amount is crucial; taking too much can have the opposite effect on brain function. Some even cause certain sensitive people to feel speedy or anxious or, with other nutrients, slow and drowsy. Just because these are naturally occurring substances doesn't mean they are free of side effects. As with any nutritional information, you should check with your physician or health care professional for dietary advice. Please read the narrative about each item *before* trying it out.

Again, it's important to experiment to see what works for you. There is no "one size fits all" rule for nutrition. Each person has a unique metabolism and reacts differently than anyone else. For example, although some of these things I consume every day, others I can't take at all because they either make me speedy or cloud my mind. I don't think they are harming me, but I simply don't like the way they make me feel. Each person needs to experiment and decide what works and what doesn't.

The Superstars: Blueberries, Omega-3s, Green Tea and Curcumin

The four most outstanding foods for stimulating neurogenesis are blueberries, omega-3 fatty acids, green tea and curcumin. It's worth considering making these a part of your regular diet.

An ode to blueberries. It's hard to sing blueberries' praises highly enough. Blueberries act in so many ways to promote neurogenesis and protect the brain from cognitive decline that if blueberries were a drug, pharmaceutical companies would be bombarding us with ads to entice us to upgrade our brain with this "miracle drug."

Numerous studies show adding blueberries to the daily diet of mice increases neurogenesis significantly. [1-3] Further, blueberries seem to protect against cognitive decline, inflammation, oxidation (free radical damage), radiation, and glycation. Generally it takes different substances to protect against any one of these things. That blueberries have so many effects is little short of astounding. Consuming about a cup a day is the equivalent human portion that animal studies have suggested.

Blueberries are packed with polyphenols, especially flavonoids called anthocyanins that stimulate neurogenesis. More specifically the anthocyanin dye, which causes the dark blue color, crosses the blood-brain barrier to stimulate neurogenesis. This anthocyanin dye is also present in black currents, blackberries, and bilberries, though these have not been studied as extensively.

Blueberries have been shown to reverse cognitive decline in both humans and animals. Mice bred to develop Alzheimer's showed improvements in memory when fed blueberries, and two neuroprotective chemicals were higher in these mice.[4,5] Humans with cognitive decline showed improvements after consuming blueberries daily.[6, 7, 131] Aside from increasing neurogenesis, blueberries allow better communication among neurons, something called signal transduction, and they also protect against brain injury, stroke, certain neurotoxins, excitotoxicity, and so may help with Parkinson's, MS, and other neurodegenerative diseases as well.[8-15, 124, 131]

An entire chapter could be written on the glories of blueberries, for they have other health benefits as well, helping with heart and cardiovascular health, colon and digestive health, cancer protection, and DNA protection.[16-19] A cup of blueberries a day may keep cognitive decline away.[106]

Studies have shown that blueberry extracts are as effective as fresh blueberries. In most animal studies it's the extract that is used. This makes daily blueberry intake possible for those who don't have access to fresh blueberries.

Omega-3s. Another neurogenesis superstar is the complex of omega-3 fatty acids, found in abundance in cold water fish, including wild Alaskan salmon, coho and sockeye salmon, black cod, sablefish, sardines, and herring. Omega-3s have been shown to dramatically increase neurogenesis and BDNF levels.

Neuroscience researcher Sandrine Thuret, Ph.D., of London's Kings College, reported a 40% increase in neurogenesis by adding omega-3's in Science Daily in 2007. Other studies have shown equally impressive gains in neurogenesis, elevated BDNF levels, increased in brain size, and neuroprotective benefits from omega-3s.[21, 27, 54]

Our brains are made up of about 60% fat. DHA, one of the most important of the omega-3s, constitutes about 30% of the brain's cerebral cortex.[26] In the ongoing tearing down, replacing, and rebuilding of our brains' cellular structures, **we want to consume high quality fats in order to continuously rebuild our brains with the best fats possible.** Omega-3s *are* the highest quality fats for brain development. A diet high in unhealthy or "bad" fats slows down neurogenesis but a diet high in healthy or "good" omega-3s increases neurogenesis to a higher level. [20] More about unhealthy fats later in this chapter.

Omega-3s work in a number of ways besides increasing neurogenesis. They build up bigger, more functional brains by increasing neurite growth, enhancing neuronal cell transmission, increasing neurotransmitter release, and protecting against inflammation and oxidation. [21-24, 133] **A startling new finding shows monkeys with an omega-3 rich diet exhibit well organized neural networks, much like human beings, whereas monkeys with a more limited omega-3 diet show far more limited neural networking.** [126] The implications of this for humans are enormous.

Omega-3s have been shown to help heal and repair traumatic brain injury. There are seven documented cases of successful healing of traumatic brain injury with high doses of omega-3s in the medical literature. "If you have a brick wall and it gets damaged, wouldn't you want to use bricks to repair it?" asked Dr. Michael Lewis, founder of the Brain Health Education and Research Institute. "By using [omega-3 fatty acids] in substantial doses, you provide the foundation for the brain to repair itself." [127]

Further, omega-3s have been shown to be as or more effective than prescription SSRI antidepressant medication in treating depression. Joseph R. Hibbeln, M.D., from the National Institute on Alcohol Abuse and Alcoholism (NIAAA) said in an interview, "The strongest evidence was found for managing major depressive symptoms, with the effect of omega-3s being at least as great, if not greater than, antidepressant medications." [24, 25, 125] This makes sense because, as noted in an earlier chapter, depression is linked to decreased neurogenesis, so increasing neurogenesis should help with depression.

Low levels of omega-3s are linked to lower IQs in children, higher rates of Alzheimer's, higher rates of cognitive decline and other cognitive impairments such as ADHD and dyslexia. [28, 29]

A report in the January 22, 2014, issue of the journal *Neurology* reveals lower brain volume and smaller hippocampus size in older adults is associated with lower omega-3 levels. Lead author James Pottala, Ph.D., concluded, "This study adds to the growing literature suggesting that higher omega-3 fatty acid tissue levels, which can be achieved by dietary changes, may hold promise for delaying cognitive aging and/or dementia."

Omega-3 fatty acids have three compounds that are most important: ALA, DHA, EPA. These three play critical roles in neuron growth, composition, and communication. It is possible to obtain one of the essential fatty acids (ALA) from vegetarian sources, generally flax oil, and the body can convert this to the other two critical fatty acids (EPA and DHA). This conversion, however, is extremely inefficient. According to the Pauling Institute at Oregon State University, 8% is converted to EPA and 0–4% is converted to DHA in healthy young men.

Some people's systems do not manage even this conversion rate, and the process deteriorates with age. This is why fish oil is recommended as the best source for omega-3s, although new sources from algae have recently appeared for vegetarians. Vegans and vegetarians have significantly lower levels of DHA in their bodies, which is a cause for concern. Supplementing with flax oil alone has shown increased EPA levels but not increased levels of the more important DHA. The newer, supplemental algae sources have, however, been shown to increase DHA levels.

When obtaining omega-3s in capsule form, it is preferable to buy molecularly distilled products, to ensure that no mercury or other heavy metal contamination is present, as well as only trace amounts or less of PCBs. Look for a high amount of DHA in the capsule as well as EPA. While this is also an expensive supplement, **there is no better financial investment than your own brain.** Many capsules are 1,000 mg (1 gram) and commonly recommended amounts are 2–4 grams a day for maintenance, 4–6 grams a day for depression.

Green tea. Green tea contains polyphenols, the most powerful of which is epigallocatechin gallate (EGCG), a type of catechin. Green tea's polyphenols have been shown to increase neurogenesis, BDNF levels, and to have strong health benefits ranging from cancer prevention to fat loss, plus cardiovascular benefits, immunity improvement, and glucose reduction. [30-33] ECGC and green tea's other polyphenols not only increase neurogenesis but, like blueberries and omega-3s, exert powerful antioxidant and anti-inflammatory effects as well. Green tea has clear cognitive benefits and even improves working memory, which is one of the most difficult functions to increase. [145]

It's important to remember that although green tea has less caffeine than regular tea, usually half or a third as much, this amount is still stimulating, although it may seem less so because of L-theanine, one of the polyphenols present in green tea that produces relaxation and also increases BDNF levels. Some people like and want caffeine stimulation while others do not. For those who are sensitive to caffeine or want to avoid it, caffeine-free green tea extracts are available. Look for extracts standardized to at least 40% polyphenols, or even better, 98% polyphenols with 75% catechins and 45% ECGC.

Suggested amounts are 300–1,000 mg daily without caffeine. Higher amounts with caffeine should be monitored for overstimulation. Also, chronic caffeine intake, even in low doses, decreases neurogenesis, so eliminating or reducing caffeine is advised. [34, 35] You want the equivalent of 3–10 cups of green tea daily but not the equivalent amount of caffeine.

Curcumin. Curcumin provides the yellow color in the curry spice turmeric. It has strong neurogenic effects. In addition it is a powerful anti-inflammatory and antioxidant compound. Aging populations who consume curcumin show better cognitive performance. [36, 37] It reduces beta-amyloid and plaque formation in aging humans and has high potential as part of an anti-Alzheimer's strategy. It has also shown strong antidepressant effects, which naturally follow from decreasing inflammation and increasing neurogenesis. [38]

Here again, like so many things, more is not necessarily better. Too little and there is no effect, but extremely high doses, on the other hand, appear to be toxic to cells. [36] Some people report feeling an analgesic numbness with too much. Just the right, moderate amount bestows highly beneficial effects on the brain, BDNF levels, and neurogenesis. Typical amounts are 200–1,200 mg daily, so experiment to see what's right for you.

Because it is poorly absorbed, there are several ways to enhance this. One is to make smaller particles (submicron dispersion technology). Another is to add piperine (a pepper extract) or phospholipids such as lecithin to enhance bioavailability. Research has shown not only increased absorption but also additional antidepressant effects when these are added. Piperine or lecithin can be added to a curcumin or turmeric supplement for little additional cost.

Other Foods and Nutrients that Increase Neurogenesis

The four foods above merit special attention for their neurogenesis- and brain health–promoting benefits, but there are numerous other nutrients that increase neurogenesis and BDNF levels. Since these often work via different metabolic pathways, eating a variety of foods that activate the brain from multiple directions is probably wiser than relying on a single source.

As with the four superstars above, whole chapters could be devoted to each of these nutrients. What follows is just a short summary of research on these nutrients and standard suggested dosages. The interested reader should consult PubMed for more information.

Whole soy foods such as tofu, edamame, soy milk, soy nuts, as well as soy isoflavone extracts containing daidzein and genistein. Soy has been shown to be neuroprotective. Key extracts, particularly daidzein and genistein, have been shown to increase neurogenesis. [42] It is believed that that the isoflavones present in soy mimic estrogen, and estrogen has also been shown to increase neurogenesis. This is true for naturally occurring estrogen, but not for non-bioidentical hormones such as Premarin, which decrease neurogenesis. [43-45]

Because of the increase in estrogenic compounds from soy intake, men should exercise caution with soy and soy extracts. Some males have reported decreased sex drive with soy or soy extract use. Testosterone, like estrogen, has been shown to promote neurogenesis, and it appears that both male and female sex hormones are equally neurogenic. [46-49]

Ginseng extract. Ginseng has been shown to increase neurogenesis, protect the brain from injury and stroke, enhance memory, and have antidepressant effects. [50-53] This herb causes some people to feel overstimulated though, so just because it's good for you doesn't mean it's right for you. As with all information in this book, each person must make his or her own determination.

Ginkgo biloba. This has been hailed as a memory booster for some years now. While a few studies failed to show improvements in patients with dementia, other studies have confirmed cognitive and memory improvements. Research shows it does increase neurogenesis, raise BDNF levels, and enhance cognitive function, as well as reducing amyloid beta plaque in Alzheimer's sufferers. [57, 58, 63, 93] Recommended dose is usually about 120 mg per day of standardized extract.

Quercetin. This flavonoid is widely found in many fruits and vegetables. It increases neurogenesis and BDNF levels, and it has anti-inflammatory, antioxidant, and other beneficial health effects. Standard dose is 500 mg, once or twice daily. [57, 93]

Vitamin E. In large doses vitamin E promotes neurogenesis. Paradoxically, vitamin E deficiency also promotes neurogenesis. [59] This makes sense given that mild or acute stress can increase neurogenesis, while stronger or chronic stress slows neurogenesis. Vitamin E has many other health benefits for heart health, cancer, eye health, and as a general antioxidant, so it is a helpful vitamin to consider including in your diet. Much research has found that the gamma form is more potent and preferable when choosing a supplement. A mix of forms is suggested, with effective doses ranging from 200–800 IU per day.

Piperine. This extract from pepper appears with many supplements because of its ability to increase absorption of such things as curcumin. It also increases neurogenesis and BDNF levels in higher amounts. [86] Standard dose is 95% extract, 10 mg once or twice daily.

DHEA and pregnenolone. Pregnenolone is a precursor to DHEA, which in turn is a precursor to testosterone, estrogen, and other androgens. Both are called "youth hormones" because levels decline with age. In large amounts they increase neurogenesis and may be neuroprotective for Alzheimer's sufferers. [89, 90] Usual doses are low, 10–100 mg daily.

Tryptophan and 5-HTP. Tryptophan and 5-HTP are chemical precursors to serotonin, and increased serotonin levels appear to promote neurogenesis. [63] As noted earlier it seems that increased neurogenesis rather than serotonin leads to antidepressant effects. Tryptophan can also be used as a sleep aid. Doses for tryptophan are usually 500–1,000 mg for 5-HTP, usually 50–300 mg, one to three times daily.

Rhodiola. This herbal adaptogen from Siberia has alkaloids that stimulate neurogenesis. Because it is stimulating, it is best taken in the morning rather than the evening, and sensitive individuals may want to avoid it. [64]

Melatonin. This hormone secreted by the pineal gland has long been known to have health benefits. The body secretes melatonin at night, when it's dark and we're asleep. Levels drop as we age, as does neurogenesis, and, accordingly, sleep disturbances increase. Melatonin increases neurogenesis and helps regulate it. [66-68,146] It also increases the immune system's capacity and has anti-cancer effects. Melatonin can be used as a sleep aid at night. Here again there is wide individual variation: some people take 1 mg per night while others take 20–30 mg per night. This is a vivid example of how you need to individualize your own approach to brain health.

Mulberry. This plant has long been used in traditional Oriental medicine, and it has been shown to stimulate neurogenesis. [69] Standardized extract 500 mg daily.

Red Sage, aka danshen and salvia. This plant also has a long history in traditional Oriental medicine, especially for stroke recovery. It has been shown to have a strong effect in increasing neurogenesis. [70] Available as a 60% extract, 1,000 mg (1 gram), twice daily is usually recommended.

Goji berry, aka wolfberry. This tasty dried berry from the Himalayas has been known for its powerful antioxidant properties, but it has now been confirmed that it has strong neurogenesis-stimulating effects as well as enhancing sexual performance. The pro-sexual effects are believed to be related to the increase in neurogenesis. [71, 75] Available as dried berries or as a 60% standardized extract, 500 mg, once or twice daily.

Grape seed extract. This compound, which is beneficial for the heart and circulatory system, has been shown to increase neurogenesis. [73] Available as an extract standardized to 90% polyphenols, 100 mg, once or twice daily. Some people find this stimulating.

Lotus root extract. The lotus flower is one of the East's most sacred plants. An extract of the lotus root has been shown to promote neurogenesis. [74] It is not commercially available at the time of this writing but hopefully will be soon.

St. John's wort. This herb has been demonstrated to be effective against depression. Some studies show it to be more effective than SSRIs for mild to moderate depression and it has fewer side effects. It is used more widely in Europe than in the United States, where it is a prescription medication. It increases neurogenesis and BDNF levels. [96, 98] Standardized extract taken once or twice a day depending on dosage.

Apigenin. This is a little known compound present in many fruits and vegetables such as grapefruit, celery, and parsley. It has been shown to induce neurogenesis. [99] Standard dose is 50 mg, once or twice daily.

Lithium. This mineral is used in the treatment of bi-polar disorder in large amounts and has shown neuroprotective benefits from the brain shrinkage caused by the disorder. It increases BDNF levels in the brain. It can also be taken in small (e.g., 5 mg) amounts, but some people find it makes them relaxed or sleepy, even at these small amounts, so be careful if you experiment with this. [65, 80, 81]

Hesperidin. This flavonoid is found widely in fruits and vegetables and has been shown to increase the rate of neurogenesis by 25–41%. With most nutrients we don't yet know if the neurogenesis increase is due to greater neuron birth or survival. With hesperidin we do know. It comes via an increase in the survival rate of neural progenitor cells. Thus, like an enriched environment, it functions to keep alive the newborn neurons rather than having them die off early on. [130]

Hopefully in the near future, as research in this area enlarges its scope, we will know more precisely which nutrients increase the number of new neurons, which ones increase the survival rates, and which ones do both, with percentages for each. Dosages vary in supplements from 100–500 mg.

Luteolin. This compound from peanuts has strong anti-inflammatory and antidepressant effects on the brain as well as increases neurogenesis and BDNF. [97, 100, 103] The usual amount in many formulations is too small to have much effect, but 50–200 mg daily is more effective.

Science Moves Forward

The nutrients and herbs discussed above have been shown to increase neurogenesis. There are also medications that increase neurogenesis. These include: the antidepressants SSRIs, SNRIs,

NRIs, MAOIs; the diabetes drug metformin; [72, 74] and the Alzheimer's medications tacrine, galantamine or memantine. [104] There are others, but the focus of this book is on naturally occurring foods and nutrients rather than prescription medications.

Within a few years I imagine both lists will double, but this is what the science shows for now. The next section contains nutrients that increase BDNF or other neurotrophins and may in the future be shown to increase neurogenesis.

Foods and Nutrients that Increase BDNF and May Increase Neurogenesis

Magnesium-L-threonate. Brain levels of magnesium are correlated with cognitive performance. Most people are deficient in magnesium, even some who take supplemental magnesium, since it does not pass the blood-brain barrier very well. A new form of magnesium developed at the Massachusetts Institute of Technology (MIT) called magnesium-L-threonate has been shown to significantly increase magnesium levels in the brain, boost cognitive performance, increase BDNF levels, and prevent Alzheimer's cognitive decline in mice. [78, 79] Usual dose is 2,000 mg daily (three capsules).

Beta-alanine and L-carnosine. Beta-alanine is an amino acid precursor to L-carnosine, which is a powerful anti-glycating agent and antioxidant. Beta-alanine is a much cheaper way to increase carnosine levels in the blood and brain. It increases BDNF levels and may have anti-anxiety effects as well. [82, 83] Usual dose is 1,000 mg (1 gram) of beta-alanine or 500 mg of L-carnosine, once or twice daily.

Vitamin D. It is known both as the "sunshine vitamin" and the "happiness vitamin," but vitamin D deficiency is still widespread.

It is an antioxidant, anti-inflammatory, and neuroprotective. Vitamin D increases BDNF levels and has been shown to help with depression, even forms of depression not linked to seasonal affective disorder (SAD.) Low levels of vitamin D are linked to depression, diabetes, and dementia. [84, 144] The August 6 edition of Science Daily reported on a comprehensive, six-year long study that concluded, "Our results confirm that vitamin D deficiency is associated with a substantially increased risk of all-cause dementia and Alzheimer's disease." It is very difficult to get enough from diet alone unless you spend a lot of time in the sun. Blood tests can show your level, with ideal ranges between 50-70 ng/ml, or 125-175 nmol/L. Usual dose is 3,000–5,000 IU daily.

Magnolol. This is an extract derived from magnolia bark and has been used in Chinese medicine to treat depression. It increases BDNF levels and may be protective against the amyloid B plaque in Alzheimer's. [85] It also appears to reduce the stress hormone cortisol, and since cortisol levels increase with age, this compound or other strategies for reducing cortisol are helpful in aging. Reducing cortisol in itself upregulates neurogenesis. It comes as an extract of 90%, 200 mg, once or more daily, or as a patented product called Relora.

Alpha lipoic acid (ALA). This antioxidant also increases BDNF levels. [76] Usual dosage ranges are 50–300 mg, once or twice a day. This nutrient is stimulating for some people, so exercise caution with dosage level.

Ashwagandha. This is an Indian herb long praised for its regenerative powers. It increases dendrite growth and has demonstrated antidepressant, neuroprotective, and cognitive-enhancing effects. [39-41] Studies suggest it increases neurogenesis, and while definitive experiments have not yet been carried out to confirm this, we do know BDNF levels are increased. Doses depend on the concentration of the particular extract, but 5–8% extracts are commonly taken once or twice daily.

Resveratrol. The research has been mixed on this compound. Because it mimics some of the effects of caloric restriction some researchers have assumed it would therefore promote neurogenesis. Studies show conflicting results, however, some show neurogenesis is inhibited, others show neurogenesis is promoted. The initial enthusiasm over resveratrol's health benefits has given way to more limited results, mainly for overweight or ill subjects rather than normals. Some people feel spacey taking resveratrol, so you should find out for yourself. Many people have adopted a "wait and see" attitude until future research sorts this out. [60, 61] Doses vary from 20–400 mg daily.

Cocoa flavonoids and chocolate. While there have been numerous claims made that chocolate and the flavonoids found in cocoa increase neurogenesis, at the time of this publication it has not been shown to be true, although BDNF levels are affected positively. [77] While some studies have failed to show any cognitive effects, two studies did show cognitive improvements and several have shown mood improvements. [55, 56] The flavonoids in cocoa demonstrate health benefits for the heart and vascular system, and this may in turn help brain function. One drawback is that cocoa comes with the stimulant theobromine, a close relative of caffeine, which may impair neurogenesis along similar pathways that caffeine does.

Milk thistle extract. This herbal extract, also known as silymarin, is widely used for its beneficial effects on the liver. It also is neuroprotective. Although it does not appear to increase BDNF, it does increase NGF and promotes neurite growth. [87] Usual doses are 300 mg, once or twice daily.

Pantethine. This is a precursor to the vitamin B5, but its action is believed to occur along other pathways. It increases BDNF, has antidepressant effects and it helps bring about healthy cholesterol levels. [88] Usual dose is 50–500 mg daily.

Huperzine A. This is another extract from a Chinese herb that has neuroprotective effects and increases BDNF levels. [91, 92] Usual doses are 200–800 mcg, once or twice daily. This has also shown promise as an Alzheimer's treatment as it also increases a neurotransmitter involved in memory, acetylcholine.

Phosphatidylserine. This compound is produced by the brain to build new brain cells. Levels decrease as we age, and it is available as a supplement in the US (in Europe it is by prescription only). It is effective in enhancing memory in older adults, has shown antidepressant effects, and it increases BDNF levels. [101, 102] Doses range from 100 mg daily for memory enhancement to 300 mg for antidepressant effects. In higher doses it can be stimulating, which may contribute to its antidepressant effects.

Cinnamon. This flavorful spice upregulates BDNF as well as another neurotrophin (NT-3), but taking pure cinnamon can be toxic. [105] It's better to take a cinnamon extract that has removed the toxins. Doses vary depending upon the extract.

A Neurohealthy Diet to Promote Neurogenesis

Okay, so we can't just eat a diet of curried salmon, blueberries, and green tea. We need a variety of nutritious foods. So what to eat to support neurogenesis and brain health?

Many people are feeling a kind of "intellectual whiplash" from the contradictory messages about food coming at us from the media. Should I eat low fat or high fat? High carb or low carb? What about protein? What about vitamins? Raw or cooked?

GMO or non-GMO? Organic or not? Grass-fed or grain-fed beef? Is gluten harmful or are the dangers overblown? Should I eat many small meals or a few bigger meals? With so many authorities saying such contradictory things, it's hard not to be confused.

This section could occupy a book in itself, actually several. But rather than drag you through more than you want to know, **I'd like to boil this discussion down to the key points in a few easy to digest pages.**

This is the very essence of what you need to know for neurohealthy eating, so you'll be able to pick and choose neurogenic foods and avoid neurotoxic foods wherever you are. Readers who want to delve into this more deeply are encouraged to read some of the excellent resources out there, including *Why We Get Fat* by Gary Taubes, *Cholesterol Is Not the Culprit* by Fred Kummerow, M.D., *The Big Fat Surprise* by Nina Teicholz and the YouTube video *Sugar: The Bitter Truth* by Robert Lustig, M.D.

Diet, like science itself, is a moving target. What science declares as healthy in one era can be changed or reversed in another. Usually this is seen as science was wrong and now it's right. Sometimes this is the case. More often, however, this change reflects a growing understanding that more closely approximates the facts.

For example, the dietary guidelines in place since the 1960s are shifting from high carbohydrate, low fat recommendations to **current recommendations for lower carbohydrates and more healthy fats.** Based on the flawed research of Ancel Keys, M.D., in the 1950s, conventional medicine long believed that fat, especially saturated fat, was responsible for heart disease and obesity, and saturated fat should be limited to 10% of calories. Carbohydrates were better for the body and should be 60% of calories.

However, the latest research shows this isn't true. Even *Time* magazine, an exemplar of accepted, conventional medical advice, declared that science had been incorrect in a cover article called "Eat Butter: Scientists labeled fat the enemy. They were wrong" (June 12, 2014.) **Excess carbohydrates are the real culprit in heart disease and obesity, not dietary fat.**

The obesity and heart disease epidemic began after Americans and the world started to follow the low fat/high carb dietary guidelines. Flawed medical and dietary advice made the very problems it was trying to help much worse and resulted in a massive health epidemic for much of the modern world.

One reading of this is: first science was wrong and now it's right. A more nuanced version would be: science seized on a partial truth about fats and ran with it. **Now a more complete picture is emerging, some fats are indeed unhealthy (or "bad") while others are healthy (or "good").** We now know lumping all fats together was a mistake, though understandable given the limited view at the time.

There is currently a better, more inclusive understanding that revises this earlier message that all fat is bad. Science erred in thinking it had the whole truth when it had only grasped a part of it. Science's understanding will always be partial and therefore will always be evolving.

Food for Thought

Before going into specifics, it's worth mentioning one approach to diet called caloric restriction (CR), where all nutrients are taken in but only 30–40% of calories are consumed. This results in increased neurogenesis. Because it means feeling hungry much of the time, however, it's not a viable, long-term option for most people. This chapter focuses on strategies that are easily available and doable. **However, it's worth noting that the opposite—excess calories, unhealthy fats, and sugar—reduce neurogenesis.** Try to avoid overeating, especially unhealthy fats and sugar in all forms.

Recently a more tolerable form of CR, called intermittent fasting, has become popular. It comes in different varieties. One popular approach involves eating 25% of normal calories two days a week, which is about 600 calories for men and 500 for women, and then eating normally the other five days (the 5:2 diet). Some people abstain from food altogether for one or two days a week. Another approach is to limit food intake to an 8-10 hour window each day (say between 10 AM and 6 PM), which also triggers the body's adaptive response to use fats as fuel rather than only glucose. Recent research shows weight loss when not eating for 12-14 hours each day but weight gain when eating anytime, even when the same number of calories are consumed.

Intermittent fasting more closely approximates the evolutionary past where our cavemen and cavewomen ancestors toggled between periods of plenty and periods with little or no food. **During these periods of no food, the body repairs itself, and, as in times of short term stress, increases neurogenesis.** It's as if the body signals the brain to wake up and think hard to figure out a way to get out of this stress.

Intermittent fasting will not become a lifestyle for most people, although restricting eating to an 8 or 10 or 12-hour window may become more popular as its benefits become known. However, what is most important is learning to eat in an ongoing, neurohealthy way.

Neurohealthy Eating In a Nutshell

The core of a neurohealthy diet is this:

a diet high in healthy fats that is anti-inflammatory, low-glycemic, high fiber, and antioxidant rich promotes neurogenesis. It will have lots of non-starchy vegetables and low glycemic fruits, grass-fed meats, and wild fish, pasture-raised eggs and dairy, with little to no processed, fried, or pro-inflammatory foods, unhealthy fats or high glycemic foods (sugar, simple carbs, starchy vegetables).

Let's unpack this a little more.

There are four key areas that guide this discussion:

- fats (healthy and unhealthy)
- sugar, carbohydrates, and the damage of glycation
- oxidation
- chronic inflammation

All four areas are intertwined. Let's first look at them separately, then see how they interact. Once you understand this, a neurohealthy approach to eating falls into place.

We begin with some words of caution. First, some of what you read here may conflict with what you may believe about a good diet, and some of it may conflict with other studies about enhancing certain functions. For example, while caffeine may improve certain kinds of memory performance in the short run, it decreases neurogenesis. **Each of us must choose for ourselves what we do to our brain.** Second, since diet and science are moving targets, even these guidelines will be refined further as science continues to advance.

The Evolutionary Context

Any discussion of diet needs to include the evolutionary context that human beings developed in. For hundreds of millions of years our ancient animal predecessors, followed by mammals, then primates and then early humans, evolved by eating what was available—wild plants, meat, and fish.

Our hunter-gatherer forefathers and foremothers appeared in the form of modern humans about 50,000 years ago. **For the first 250,000 years our ancestors hunted and gathered plants, roots, vegetables, nuts, and fruits.** Sugar, in the form of fruit, was rarely available, mostly in late summer, when it was advantageous to store a little fat for the coming winter.

Agriculture developed only about 10,000 years ago, a blink of the eye in genetic time, and agriculture dramatically changed how humans ate. Suddenly grains (and carbohydrates) became readily available, although sugar and processed foods didn't appear on the scene in the massive quantities we see today until the last 30–50 years.

Many estimates have been done on how our hunter-gatherer ancestors ate, and these estimates are roughly similar.

Note the contrast with current dietary guidelines:

Hunter-gatherers: 60–75% fat, about 20% protein, about 5–20% carbohydrates.
Government guidelines: 60% carbohydrates, 20% protein, and 20% fat.

Notice how fats and carbs are reversed in a modern diet. Healthy, high quality fats were our main source of energy for millions and millions of years. **Our bodies were never designed to deal with the massive onslaught of sugar and carbohydrates that make up today's average diet.** Of course there will be blowback. The epidemics of diabetes, obesity, metabolic syndrome, heart disease, inflammation, cognitive decline, and Alzheimer's are some of what results.

We want to eat in alignment with what our bodies evolved to live on. When we change our diets this drastically, we're fooling with Mother Nature. And Mother Nature has the final say in these matters, not the human ego.

Fats

We've been led to believe the following fat myths:

- Eating fat makes us fat.
- Fat is bad, fat clogs our arteries and causes heart disease.
- Saturated fat (especially animal fat) is the worst, but all fat is bad.
- Carbs are good, keep us thin, and are healthy.

These myths will take time to die.

When false information like this has been drilled into you for most of your life, it takes a while to shake loose from these prejudices. Layer after layer of conditioning needs to be shed so you can make a real change. **Give yourself time to fully let in a more complete understanding of diet than conventional advice has suggested over the past few decades.**

"Feed Your Head"

In an earlier section on Heraclitus's brain it was explained how the brain is in constant movement. Every single day and night of our lives our brains are continually tearing down and pruning unused synapses and neural networks, modeling and remodeling neural structures, producing new neurons and building new synaptic connections. The brain is always "under construction." **This ongoing construction project requires high quality building materials, mostly in the form of good, healthy fats.**

Just as athletes need plenty of good, high quality protein to build up muscles, everyone needs lots of good, high quality fats to build up the brain— continuously, for this is an ongoing process— day in and day out. Jefferson Airplane got it right when they sang, "Feed your head."

Fats (technically fatty acids) make up 60% of the brain's solid matter. DHA and cholesterol are two key players. About a third of the brain's fat consists of the omega-3 fatty acid DHA. Although the brain has only 2% of the body's weight, it has 25% of its cholesterol.

Healthy Fats

What makes a fat healthy or "good"? Healthy fat provides building material for the brain, nerves, and body, as well as being a source of energy. Good, high quality fats build neurons and glial cells that operate efficiently, with greater energy and capacity for signal transmission. Better cognition, better memory, faster learning, and greater resistance to stress and depression are all associated with a diet of high quality fats.

Omega-3s are probably the single most important nutrient we need for brain health. Not only do omega-3 fatty acids promote neurogenesis, they provide the raw materials for neuronal growth, as the earlier section on omega-3s explains.

Less well known is the role of cholesterol. It is essential for synapses to form, for the myelin sheaths that protect neurons, and for communication between neurons and energy. Cholesterol also is necessary to produce the glucocorticoid hormones that regulate glucose, DHEA, the sex hormones testosterone and estrogen, and it's a precursor to vitamin D, all of which are essential for good brain function.

With low cholesterol, brain function declines, neurite growth is disrupted, plus new learning and memory are impaired. **Cholesterol is an essential nutrient of the brain.** [133]

It's probably a surprise to discover that healthy fat, including cholesterol, is our ally. Cholesterol in particular has been so thoroughly demonized that it can be hard to believe how important it is for health and good brain function.

In study after study, cholesterol is getting rehabilitated and appreciated for its essential role in brain function. For example, the famous Framingham Heart Study did rigorous cognitive testing on almost 2,000 men and women. Higher cholesterol levels were associated with higher cognitive functioning while lower levels of cholesterol were associated with poorer memory, lower scores on abstract reasoning, attention, and concentration, verbal fluency and executive function. [135]

In 2008 a study looked at healthy older adults. Memory functions were best for those with higher cholesterol levels. Those that had lower cholesterol levels fared much more poorly on cognitive tests of memory. The authors stated their conclusions simply, **"High cholesterol is associated with better memory function."** [136]

A large meta-analysis involving over 500,000 people in almost 80 different studies showed those who consume larger amounts of saturated fats have no greater risk for heart disease than those who consume less. [133]

The failure of studies in the 1950s and '60s to distinguish between cholesterol and oxidized cholesterol has resulted in an explosion of statin drugs to lower cholesterol. But memory loss, brain fog, and poor cognitive function are widespread side effects of statins. It's now clear that these side effects must occur when the body and brain don't have enough of this essential fat to function optimally. This led one nutrition researcher to declare, "Statins could kill your memory—eggs could cure it." [133]

Further, many physicians continue to fail to distinguish between types of LDL ("bad cholesterol"). Having high HDL ("good" cholesterol) is clearly healthy, but recent science shows that LDL levels alone mean very little. Distinguishing between the large, "fluffy" LDL molecules that are benign and the low density LDL molecules that pose serious health dangers is essential for determining heart and cardiovascular risk. Ask you doctor for this level of cholesterol testing rather than relying on old standards that can be misleading.

Healthy fats include:

- monosaturated fats (like olive oil, avocadoes)
- saturated fats (from grass-fed meat, pasture-raised butter, eggs, yogurt, and coconut oil)
- unsaturated omega-3s (from fish oil, flax oil, raw nuts)

Unhealthy Fats

What makes a fat unhealthy or "bad"? **Unhealthy fat clogs up our blood vessels, degrades our brain, and promotes oxidation and inflammation.** Low quality, unhealthy fats slow down the brain, limit the quality and number of new neurons, decrease signal quality, erode memory, make us more vulnerable to stress, clog our arteries, and undermine our health and brain function. Sometimes an "unhealthy" fat is simply too much of an essential fat that is healthy in smaller amounts (such as omega-6 fatty acid).

The real culprit in the misleading studies from the 1950s and '60s was actually oxidized cholesterol, not cholesterol itself. Cholesterol is necessary for good brain functioning. Cooking with vegetable oils like soy, corn, safflower, or cotton produces oxidized cholesterol that creates heart disease. The body treats oxidized cholesterol and other oxidized fat like invading bacteria. It sends macrophages after oxidized fatty acids in the bloodstream, and it is primarily this that produces the atherosclerotic plaque that narrows blood vessels and results in cardiovascular disease. When this plaque breaks loose, it can result in a stroke or a heart attack. **Oxidized cholesterol is the real culprit, not dietary cholesterol that isn't oxidized.** [149]

Another type of unhealthy fats are pro-inflammatory fats. Omega-6 fatty acids are essential nutrients that help the body mount an inflammatory response. For most of human evolution the ratio of anti-inflammatory omega-3s to pro-inflammatory omega-6s was about 1:1 or 1:2. Today's diet, by contrast, has ratios of 1:20 or 1:30. The pro-inflammatory omega-6s come to us through polyunsaturated vegetable oils such as corn, soy, safflower, cottonseed, sunflower (not olive, coconut, or canola, however) processed foods and through conventional meats and eggs.

Conventional grain-fed meat, eggs, and dairy have higher amounts of omega-6s and lower amounts of omega-3s. However, grass-fed beef and pasture-raised eggs and dairy have much higher amounts of protective omega-3s to counterbalance the omega-6s. According to a 2009 study by the USDA and Clemson University, besides having higher total omega-3s, the ratio of omega-3s to omega-6s for grass-fed beef was 1:1.65 vs. grain-fed beef's unhealthier ratio of 1:4.84. [138]

The harm from trans fats is by now quite well publicized, and there is currently a movement to take trans fats out of the food supply entirely. Trans fatty acids raise LDL cholesterol, lower the "good" HDL cholesterol, increase triglycerides in the blood and promote systemic inflammation, and increase the risk of heart disease, stroke, and type 2 diabetes. It's recently been discovered that a diet high in trans fats increases the risk of Alzheimer's. [141] It's found in many processed foods, from doughnuts, cakes, cookies, and margarine to French fries, and is often labeled as "partially hydrogenated vegetable oil."

Unhealthy fats include:

- oxidized fatty acids and cholesterol (from fried foods, burned meat, overcooked eggs, cooking with vegetable oils and foods cooked in them, as well as from high blood sugar)
- pro-inflammatory fats like omega-6 fatty acids (from vegetable oils)
- trans fat (from margarine and other processed foods)

Current thinking is that body and brain need a plentiful amount of healthy fats to function optimally. **The problems with heart disease, diabetes, metabolic syndrome, cognitive decline, and Alzheimer's appear to be connected to eating unhealthy**

fats, not healthy fats, as well as too much sugar and other high carbohydrate foods. This brings us to the second issue of sugar and glycation.

Remember the brain uses 20–30% of the body's energy, oxygen, and blood. Since it uses so much blood to transport the needed oxygen and glucose, three problems that damage the brain are glycation, oxidation, and chronic inflammation. Since all three have neurotoxic effects, minimizing these influences is essential for optimal brain health.

Sugar, carbohydrates, and glycation. In the average Western diet sugar in the form of glucose supplies most of the energy to the brain and body. As carbohydrates are broken down in the body into sugar and blood sugar levels rise, the pancreas secretes insulin, which allows the cells to utilize glucose.

Carbohydrates have soared in the diets of most people, and after each high carbohydrate meal there are glucose surges that then produce insulin spikes. When this is repeated over and over again for years, the body gets hammered with insulin, and it overwhelms the body's capacity to process sugar. This results in cells producing less insulin receptors, which is known as insulin resistance. **It's estimated that 50-80% of adults in the US have insulin resistance.**

In insulin resistance there are higher amounts of both glucose and insulin in the bloodstream. High insulin levels are harmful, but high glucose levels are even more damaging. When proteins or fats get exposed to high glucose levels they become glycated, creating advanced glycation end products (or AGEs). AGEs set off an inflammatory cascade that includes activating inflammatory genes, they in turn damage many systems throughout the body, including the heart, eyes, brain, and vascular system. **Increasing AGEs occur**

naturally with normal aging and are a major cause of dysfunction as we grow older.

When blood sugar levels rise due to insulin resistance, AGEs accumulate much more rapidly than normal, causing the cross-linking of proteins (like the browning of a chicken) and creating protease-resistant aggregates in the brain, which interfere with how neurons communicate.

Glycation changes how fatty acids function in the body so that proteins produce up to 50 times more free radicals (ROS) and LDL molecules stop transporting cholesterol to neurons and so diminish brain function. **Higher glucose levels are associated with cognitive decline as we age and brain shrinkage.** [108, 136]

Glycation leads to increasing inflammation as well as oxidation, and oxidation leads to increased glycation. As these two processes reinforce each other, they wreak havoc in the brain and body with problems ranging from diabetes and blindness to nerve and organ damage. [109]

Alzheimer's disease is being called "Type 3 diabetes" by many experts. Beginning in 2005 the theory that Alzheimer's is a form of diabetes of the brain was put forward and is now receiving increasing acceptance. Insulin resistance and faulty glucose metabolism that result from overconsuming sugar and carbohydrates may be a common root for Alzheimer's and diabetes. [137]

It is estimated that by 2020 as much as one-third of Americans will be diabetic. If this is true, over the following decades there will be a tsunami of Alzheimer's and dementia that will overwhelm the healthcare system. This diet is a way to avoid this.

Further, high glucose levels signal insulin to store the excess glucose as fat in the body. A high carbohydrate diet leads to obesity. The obesity epidemic is directly traceable to the dietary recommendations of eating more carbohydrates. **Much of the current obesity epidemic, both in the US and around the world, is now being traced to higher and higher sugar and carbohydrate intake.** The reason grain is fed to beef is to fatten them up quickly. Its effect in humans is similar.

Excess carbohydrates, especially sugar and flour, cause insulin to signal the body to store this excess by converting it to fat, which in turn decreases neurogenesis as well as being associated with lower brain volume. [110] In one experiment neurogenesis was cut almost in half on a high sugar diet. The implications for children, diet, and brain health are staggering. But for adults also, high sugar intake is bad for both body and brain. **Shifting to a diet that has more protein and healthy fats while decreasing sugar and carbohydrates is rapidly gaining research support.** [128, 129]

To prevent this or slow it down means eating low glycemic foods, that is foods that convert their energy to sugar slowly (low glycemic index) and have a low amount of total carbohydrate or sugar calories (low glycemic load). It also means avoiding foods that contain a lot of AGEs, for eating AGEs is damaging to the body, just as forming them internally is. Frying, grilling, and roasting all produce glycation and glycotoxins. Low-temperature cooking is better for the brain—poaching, steaming, baking at low temperatures.

Oxidation. One natural result of oxygen metabolism is the creation of reactive oxygen species (ROS) that are highly damaging to cell structures. Rust is oxidized iron, and the brown color that forms on an apple slice is also the result of oxidation.

Normally the body neutralizes these through its own antioxidant defenses. But without proper nutritional support the body's defenses get overwhelmed. **The result is oxidative**

stress that tears down cells and produces inflammation, cancer, cardiovascular disease, lowered neurogenesis, and even brain cell death.

Cooking at high temperatures also produces oxidation. When foods are fried, grilled, or processed (such as margarine, powdered egg yolk, or powdered milk) they are subjected to high temperatures that oxidize fats.

A recent study showed that people who ate baked or broiled fish at least once a week had 14% more gray matter in the part of the brain responsible for cognition and 4% greater volume in the memory area. However, people who ate fried fish had no such benefit. [142] Eating fried fish also increases the risk of heart failure. [143]

Cooking with most vegetable oils produces oxidized fats at an alarming rate. The vegetable oil industry jumped on the low saturated fat bandwagon in the 1960s, donating vast sums of money to the American Heart Association. It's one of the bitterest ironies of the modern era that the dietary guidelines of the American Heart Association for low fat and high carbohydrates helped create the very epidemic of heart disease they were attempting to prevent.

What wasn't known at the time is how corn oil, sunflower, soy, safflower, cottonseed, and canola oil oxidize at low levels of heat and create trans fats that are toxic. Even olive oil becomes oxidized and rancid when cooking at only slightly higher temperatures and is best consumed cold, as in salad dressing. **Butter, lard, and coconut oils are far better for cooking, since these saturated fats don't oxidize at higher temperatures.**

A diet rich in antioxidants includes fresh fruits and vegetables as well as supplemental vitamins C, E, A, and other carotenoids including astaxanthin, lipoic acid, NAC (a precursor to glutathione, one of the body's most important free radical scavengers), and ubiquinol (Co-Q 10). Much research still needs to be done on the impact of nutrition on brain health. Vitamin E, for example, is composed of eight different substances, four tocopherols and four tocotrienols (alpha, beta, gamma, delta forms of each). Each has different effects from the others. Less than 1% of the research has been done on the tocotrienols, even though alpha-tocotrienol appears to have the greatest neuroprotective effect. [107, 148]

By now there is so much evidence that people with higher dietary levels of antioxidants are healthier and live longer than those with lower levels that it is surprising controversy still lingers in some quarters. There are many foods that are abundant in antioxidants as well as lots of extracts from plants that have high antioxidant content, such as polyphenols, flavonoids, and carotenoids. Colorful foods tend to be high in these, so eating a rainbow diet of reds, blues, purples, yellows, and greens is recommended.

Chronic inflammation. Chronic inflammation dramatically slows neurogenesis and decreases BDNF. One way chronic inflammation speeds aging is by clogging, weakening, and stiffening blood vessels. When some part of the lining of the blood vessels (endothelium) ruptures to cause bleeding or falls off to create a blockage, the result can be a heart attack or stroke.

A healthy brain needs a healthy blood supply, but chronic inflammation "chews up" the insides of our blood vessels, compromising needed blood flow. Chronic inflammation also attacks neurons and damages the brain directly. Shifting to an anti-inflammatory diet means including more foods and supplements that quench the fires of inflammation while keeping pro-inflammatory foods to a minimum. A later chapter ("Increase

Neurogenesis by Not Slowing It Down") goes into greater detail on the dangers of chronic inflammation.

There is a lot of information available online about eating an anti-inflammatory diet. **In general this means eating fresh fruits and vegetables, fish and other foods rich in omega-3s like nuts, fiber, grass-fed beef and dairy, and anti-inflammatory herbs such as ginger and garlic.**

The other side involves avoiding or reducing pro-inflammatory foods. High glycemic foods are associated with an increase in pro-inflammatory markers and are yet another reason to minimize them, especially sugar and sugar drinks such as colas or fruit juices as well as other carbohydrates. This also means minimizing omega-6s—especially trans fats which are particularly pro-inflammatory.

There are a number of helpful anti-inflammatory herbs and nutrients. Aside from the all-stars of curcumin, green tea, blueberries, and omega-3s, these include:

- ginger
- borage oil or evening primrose oil (which contain gamma-linolenic acid, or GLA)
- rosemarinic acid found in the herbs rosemary, basil, peppermint, oregano
- black cumin seed oil
- tart cherry extract
- nettle root extract
- benfotiamine
- carnosine
- fisetin

General Principles of a Neurohealthy Diet

It's been noticed by many researchers that a brain healthy diet is very similar to a heart healthy diet. But a neurohealthy diet is not only good for your heart, it also protects against stress, depression, and Alzheimer's. The following principles are guidelines for eating in ways that support neurogenesis and brain health.

Plenty of fresh vegetables and fruits. The best vegetables are those that are non-starchy (low carbohydrate content) with high amounts of fiber. Fiber gives us a "full" feeling and keeps the intestinal tract moving. Low glycemic fresh fruits, raw, fresh vegetables in salads and cooked vegetables (not overcooked) should provide the bulk of our food.

High quality fats. Healthy fats ideally make up the majority of calories (although not the bulk of food due to their higher caloric content than fruits and vegetables) for most people. These include:

- omega-3s (from high quality fish high in omega-3s, avoiding those with low omega-3s or high in omega-6s or with high mercury content, flaxseed, grass-fed beef, eggs from pasture-raised chickens)
- monosaturated fats (from extra virgin olive oil, avocadoes, nuts, and seeds)
- medium chain triglycerides (from extra virgin coconut oil)
- saturated fat from (grass-fed meat, pasture-raised eggs and milk, yogurt, cheeses)

One healthy fat stands out as superior for many things: coconut oil. Organic, extra virgin coconut oil is cheap and readily available. It has been shown to improve cognition in Alzheimer's sufferers. [140] Anecdotal reports show significant improvements in some patients with even advanced Alzheimer's who ate three tablespoons a day. Its use as a possible preventative strategy for Alzheimer's is currently being studied. Some authorities are recommending 1–3 tablespoons daily as a protective strategy for cognitive decline.

Coconut oil excels as cooking oil, for it doesn't oxidize at high temperatures. Cooking with butter, or even better with clarified butter (called ghee in India) is another safe alternative to vegetable oils that go rancid at even low heat.

Reducing unhealthy fats means reducing dangerous oxidized fats, so cook at lower temperatures, do not eat burned or charred meat, overcooked or powdered eggs, or powdered milk. It also means reducing or eliminating grain-fed conventional beef, certain fish with high mercury content such as: swordfish, marlin, tilefish, shark, ahi and bigeye tuna, as well as fish high in omega-6 such as: tilapia and many farm-raised fish. Further, it involves avoiding trans fats and most vegetable oils except extra virgin olive oil, though again, this is better used cold than for cooking.

Low sugar and carbohydrate intake. Sugar is more and more being identified as the cause of the obesity epidemic. As noted earlier, high sugar reduces neurogenesis sharply, and even "high normal" blood sugar levels are linked to smaller brain volume, especially in the hippocampus, less gray matter and cognitive decline in those over 60. [111] Getting blood sugar levels down to lower ranges is important to prevent cognitive decline. But sugar is only part of the story.

All carbohydrates eventually get converted to glucose. White flour and whole wheat flour are converted into sugar in almost the same amount of time, despite whole wheat's better press. Starchy vegetables such as potatoes, rice, and yams, have a high glycemic load that also taxes our systems.

Fruits with a high fructose content are best eaten sparingly if at all. These include: mangoes, peaches, plums, persimmons, bananas, grapes, and lychees. Of course dried fruit is almost pure sugar and better avoided. Fruit juice and carrot juice are about equal to soda in sugar content and should be minimized or eliminated.

The best carbohydrates come with lots of fiber, things like summer squash, berries, carrots, string beans, kale, bok choy, broccoli, and cauliflower. When the carbohydrate comes in the fiber like this, it takes the body a while to break down the fiber and liberate the sugar, and this time lag prevents the sugar and insulin spikes responsible for insulin resistance.

Reducing carbohydrates, especially simple carbohydrates, over time can reduce and eliminate insulin resistance. Since as much as 80% of the American population has some degree of insulin resistance (which can lead to diabetes), and since higher blood sugar levels that accompany insulin resistance is associated with greater cognitive decline, getting insulin and blood glucose levels down is important. Some people benefit from a period of eating a ketogenic diet that eliminates almost all carbs and forces the body to rely on fats for energy. Intermittent fasting is another way to sensitize the body to insulin once again.

Weight loss is a by-product of this diet. Because reducing carbohydrates lowers insulin levels in the blood, and since insulin from excess carbohydrates is turned into fat by the liver, most everyone on the neurogenesis diet will lose weight, simply and easily discovering their own natural weight. This diet is:

- pro-neurogenesis
- antidepressant

- anti-Alzheimer's
- anti-obesity

Coming Into Your Own Optimal Weight

The secret of finding your own body's optimal weight is to eat to support your brain. When your brain is well nourished, your optimal body weight follows as a matter of course. Neurohealthy eating has the happy side effect of supporting your body's natural metabolism. **It's not a special "diet" requiring willpower and feeling hungry all the time.** To the contrary, eating to fullness (not overstuffed) is normal and natural.

Eating as many healthy fats (not the unhealthy, artery-clogging and inflammatory kind) as you want leads to feeling full without the weight gain that comes from excess carbohydrates. This leads naturally to your own optimal weight.

We All Have Bad Habits

Most everyone eats foods that impair neurogenesis and damage the brain's health. Given the food choices we grow up with, it's inevitable we get attached to some of these. But remember, **dietary habits are learned.** And they can be unlearned. As you move toward increasingly neurohealthy eating, remember to be kind to yourself. It's not necessary to be as pure as the driven snow. Not everyone has problems with carbohydrate metabolism, and one size does not fit all when it comes to diet. Don't demand "perfection" from yourself.

Gradually, new healthy choices can replace old ones as our tastes change over time. We can accelerate this change by simply dropping certain food choices while trying new foods. **It takes two** or three weeks for most food habits to recede and for new habits to come online.

The biggest exception to this rule is sugar. This can be a lifelong addiction for many people. Though not everyone struggles with it, we are biologically wired to prefer this taste, as experiments with babies demonstrate. Stevia is growing as a safe alternative sweetener to sugar. But aside from this, most of our food habits are just that—habits. We can develop new habits by trying new foods and discovering how good they are.

We are better off avoiding a high calorie diet. Eating too much and being obese bring about lower neurogenesis, lower brain volume, and cognitive decline. For mothers, being obese and eating a high "bad fat" diet during pregnancy even reduces neurogenesis and BDNF levels in newborns. [112-114]

Eating less and caloric restriction increase neurogenesis, as noted earlier, but almost no one wants to feel hungry all the time. The opposite, eating too much, decreases neurogenesis. So does eating frequently, even if you consume a regular amount of calories.

Increasing time between meals increases neurogenesis, as does intermittent fasting (such as eating an early dinner and a late breakfast so that you have more than 12–14 hours of fasting, as discussed earlier). If you can increase the time between meals, this raises BDNF levels and the rate of neurogenesis. [54] It also has the desirable side benefit of decreasing insulin resistance by increasing insulin sensitivity. Intermittent fasting can improve metabolic syndrome, and metabolic syndrome has been linked to cognitive decline. [139]

Alcohol and caffeine are two other substances that decrease neurogenesis. Drinking alcohol in moderation is considered in some quarters healthy for heart and brain. But it's clear from the research that **even moderate alcohol consumption reduces neurogenesis by 40%** (which is a lot) as well as BDNF levels. Further, binge drinking in puberty and adolescence reduces neurogenesis and BDNF levels dramatically with effects well into adulthood. [115-117]

There exists a whole generation of graduate students and post-doc neuroscience researchers who have sought, in vain, to show that caffeine helps neurogenesis. Most research labs virtually run on the stuff. And because caffeine does help many people focus better for certain tasks (like doing tedious experimental record keeping or housework), it has been mightily hoped that caffeine would also increase neurogenesis. But the data show otherwise.

In fact, even low and "physiologically relevant doses" of caffeine (that is, anything you can feel) reduce neurogenesis and impair memory. [118, 119] So, if you drink much caffeine, try drinking less. And if you only drink a little, try stopping. You'll adjust within a few weeks and wonder what the big deal was. Taking extra B-5 and B-12 can help, for these are psychic energizers. **Your body and brain just need to learn to wake themselves up again naturally.** And when they do, you'll hardly miss it, unless it was hiding a deeper problem such as low thyroid.

Other factors to avoid include deficiencies in zinc, vitamin A, thiamine, and folic acid (B-1 and B-9). When we're low in these vitamins and minerals, neurogenesis slows, but when we supplement or reestablish healthy levels, normal neurogenesis resumes. [54]

Interestingly, the consistency of our food has a role in neurogenesis. Soft food is the other big factor to avoid or reduce. Eating soft food (ice cream, many processed foods, puddings, Jell-O, mashed potatoes, overcooked vegetables, bananas, etc.) reduces neurogenesis and eating liquid food reduces survival of new brain cells. A solid diet consisting of foods with a harder texture that need to be chewed increases neurogenesis, BDNF, and memory. [120-122] This has implications for older adults who've lost their teeth or who may have impaired dental abilities.

It's almost as if our brains want us to bite into life, to use our teeth and mouth and physical organism to engage with the world. Whether it's exercising or walking, chewing or listening to music, looking at colors or talking to others, neurogenesis is stimulated when we are stimulated.

What We Don't Know

What we don't know vastly outweighs what we do know about neurogenesis and the brain. One intriguing recent discovery is that certain substances only increase neurogenesis on one half of the hippocampus. SSRI drugs (antidepressant medications), for example, only increase neurogenesis along the emotional side of the hippocampus but not the other side that is related to cognition and the body. Aerobic exercise, on the other hand, increases neurogenesis along the full length of the hippocampus.

No one knows what this means yet. Does increasing neurogenesis along the emotional side have any effect on cognition and memory, or does it just impact mood? What effects do these different foods and nutrients have? Do they increase neurogenesis along both sides of the brain or just one? If so, which one? Or do different nutrients stimulate neurogenesis in different parts of the hippocampus?

How effective are these various nutrients compared to each other and compared to other things that stimulate neurogenesis? That is, it would be helpful to know if blueberries increase neurogenesis by 65% or 35%, or whether eating curcumin works synergistically to increase this number or leaves it unaffected. At present we have very little idea how much of an increase these different nutrients produce, either alone or in combination.

Are there age differences in the neurogenic boost from different nutrients? Is it better to do more of one thing at one age and less at a different age? Additionally, aside from studies on omega-3s, current research also lags behind in nutritional science with studies that lump all fats together and fail to differentiate between oxidized fats, pro-inflammatory fats, trans fats, and healthy fats.

Until we know much, much more than we do now, it makes sense to increase neurogenesis along as many lines as possible so that both sides of the hippocampus will benefit. This will maximize our physical, emotional, cognitive, and spiritual health.

Future Dreams

The epidemics of diabetes, heart disease, cancer, Alzheimer's, and obesity that plague the early 21st century will have the positive effect of forcing a radical reevaluation of medicine and health. Rather than looking to chemicals in a pill to treat disease symptoms, physicians will look to underlying causes for prevention and to establish health. There will be a return to Hippocrates's maxim, "Let food be your medicine and medicine be your food," as nutrition science brings about a level of vital health and well-being for virtually the entire population.

Doctors will be called upon after an accident or to fix a broken arm but rarely for anything else. Even most bacterial and viral infections will be fought off by the strong immune systems of the populace. Healthcare spending will be a small fraction of what it was in the medieval era of the 21st century.

Nutritional guidelines and food policy will be shaped by scientists serving the public good rather than lobbyists for farmers or pharmaceutical companies. The skewing of public policy by moneyed interests will be outlawed when the epidemics they created are recognized, and the corporate-sponsored scientists for hire will disappear shortly thereafter. The new norm will be robust health into what used to be considered very old age.

Summary

The following charts summarize the contents of this chapter.

<u>Nutrients that Increase Neurogenesis</u>

- blueberries
- omega-3s
- green tea
- curcumin
- whole soy and extracts containing daidzein and genistein
- ginseng extract
- ginkgo biloba
- quercetin
- Vitamin E
- piperine
- DHEA and pregnenolone
- tryptophan and 5-HTP
- rhodiola
- melatonin
- mulberry
- red sage, aka salvia
- goji berry, aka wolfberry

- grape seed extract
- lotus root extract
- St. John's wort
- apigenin
- lithium
- luteolin

Nutrients that Increase BDNF and May Increase Neurogenesis

- magnesium-L-threonate
- beta-alanine and L-carnosine
- Vitamin D
- magnolol
- alpha lipoic acid
- ashwagandha
- resveratrol
- cocoa flavonoids and chocolate
- milk thistle extract
- pantethine
- huperzine A
- phosphatidylserine
- cinnamon

Nutrients that Decrease Neurogenesis

- high sugar, carbohydrates, and unhealthy fats
- high amounts of food (overeating)
- inflammatory foods (fried foods, processed foods, common cooking oils like safflower, soy, sunflower, corn, and cottonseed), trans fats, refined grains, sugar, conventional, feed-lot-raised meat, eggs, and dairy)

- alcohol
- caffeine
- deficiencies in vitamins A, B-1, and B-9 (thiamine and folic acid)

The essence of a neurohealthy diet is simply this: stick to a diet high in healthy fats that is anti-inflammatory, low glycemic, low carb, low in unhealthy fats, high in fiber, and rich in antioxidants.

CHAPTER 4

BODY

On the physical level many things increase neurogenesis and BDNF levels, ranging from exercising to getting enough sleep. This section spells out physical factors other than diet that stimulate neurogenesis as well as some surprising things that slow it down.

To recap the strategy: diet and body practices to increase neurogenesis are step one in a holistic, four-fold plan to develop each part of our being: body, heart, mind, spirit. Equally important is stopping or avoiding things that shrink the brain and decrease neurogenesis and BDNF levels to ensure we don't erase the gains we make.

Two powerful ways of increasing neurogenesis are diet and exercise. Research on exercise is further along than research into nutrition, so more is known about the effects of exercise alone or exercise in combination with other factors. **Exercise increases neurogenesis to four or five times the normal rate.** However, remember that only 40–60% of these new neurons survive. To boost these survival rates to close to 100% requires an enriched environment. The big question is: **what does an "enriched environment" mean for humans?**

We have some pretty good answers for this, which are integrated seamlessly into the holistic plan offered here in order to tease out the physical, emotional, mental, and spiritual dimensions to this question. First let's look at the physical aspects of an enriched environment. These are:

- exercise (certain kinds)
- touch
- sexual experience
- sleep (7 or 8 hours per night)
- doing new things, being in novel environments, new sensory stimulation
- music, silence, natural sounds
- nature

Emily

Emily was in her late fifties and held an administrative position that kept her sitting in front of a computer for most of her days. She entered therapy concerned about feeling sluggish in her life and harboring a growing suspicion that she was slipping into depression, though she tried to maintain a positive and upbeat attitude about life.

A holistic assessment of her situation revealed that she was doing a lot of things right: she had a spiritual practice, her work at a nonprofit was meaningful, she was satisfied in her marriage, and had a strong support system of friends who loved her. But there was a way she held herself back, a long-held pattern that reflected early childhood fears about expressing herself. Her held-in energy seemed physical as well. She spoke of never enjoying PE as a child or even exercising. Though not fat, her body tissue seemed almost spongy or doughy.

"Exercise is the last thing in the world I'll do," she declared matter-of-factly as we discussed this. "I walk some around the neighborhood. I can't imagine doing more."

We worked with her childhood wounding as it manifested in her current life and along the way I gently encouraged her to try moving faster on her walks. As she reported a slight stimulation from this, I suggested she try something more strenuous. She balked at first but then agreed to give it a go. After trying out different exercise routines, she settled on aerobic dancing for an hour most mornings of the week. The first month she was miserable. But then she started getting stronger. This encouraged her to keep with it.

After eight months of regular aerobic dance classes, Emily looked and felt 20 years younger. "I've never felt this good in my life," she shared one week. "I can't even imagine getting depressed anymore. And I have more energy for other things I've thought about doing but never had the energy for. How can exercise make such a dramatic difference in my life? Everyone should know about this!"

It's true. Exercise is the single most important thing you can do for your brain and your health, far better than any pill or magic potion. So let's begin here.

Exercise

Our bodies were made to move. Evolution has shaped our bodies and selected those who could stand, walk, and run. Our hunter-gatherer ancestors were always on the move. They didn't have the luxury of sitting around for hours on end if they wanted to survive. Natural selection rewarded those who kept on the move and this primed us for movement.

Sitting for 8–12 hours a day is an extremely recent development that goes against our long evolutionary history. When we move, our brains wake up and neurogenesis increases. Sitting for long periods weakens our brains along with our bodies.

When you put a running wheel into a mouse's cage, the mouse voluntarily spends time each day running on it. **The result is that the hippocampus fairly explodes with new neurons.** By contrast, a sedentary mouse without a running wheel shows no increase in neurogenesis. [1, 3]

In terms of neurogenesis, are all forms of exercise created equal? Exercise physiologists and researchers have found that there are big differences in the type of exercise and the effects on the brain and body. **Aerobic exercise is best for neurogenesis.** The word "aerobic" means "living in air," so any exercise that uses oxygen at a high rate is an aerobic exercise. Whether it's running, walking briskly, cycling, aerobic dancing, swimming, water running, using stair climbers or ellipticals, cardio classes, soccer, tennis, hiking up a mountain, or whatever else gets you breathing fast and hard is aerobic.

Aerobic exercise can be contrasted to weight bearing exercise, that strengthens muscles (like weight lifting), or stretching exercise, that increases flexibility (like yoga or tai chi). Although weight bearing and stretching exercise have health benefits, they don't seem to increase neurogenesis. **Hence our focus on aerobic exercise, since this is the key to growing new brain cells.** [4-6, 20, 21]

Aerobic exercise reduces a brain protein called BMP (for bone morphogenetic protein) that slows down neurogenesis and keeps neural stem cells in a kind of cellular sleep. High levels of BMP slow the brain down. But according to a report in the *New York Times* (7/7/2010) just one week of mice using running wheels reduced BMP by 50%. This aerobic exercise also increased another wonderfully named protein called Noggin, which stimulates neurogenesis. Mice whose brains were infused with Noggin became, according to senior researcher Dr. Jack Kessler, "little mouse geniuses, if there is such a thing." **These mice breezed through the mouse intelligence tests and mazes they were given.**

Aerobic exercise also accelerates the heart so blood gets pumped throughout the body. Increased blood flow is one of the requirements for neurogenesis. When new brain cells develop they require blood supplies to help them grow. In fact one indication that neurogenesis is occurring is increased blood flow as measured through neuroimaging.

Aerobic exercise has positive effects beyond increasing blood flow, including anti-inflammatory, antioxidant, and hormonal changes, all of which help brain function. Beginning aerobic exercise in middle age stops the age-related decline in neurogenesis, keeps BDNF levels high, and improves memory. [22] One recent study published in *Frontiers of Aging* Neuroscience (May, 2014) showed that exercise protected those most at risk for Alzheimer's disease (with the e4 gene) and prevented both memory loss and the hippocampal shrinkage that non-exercisers showed.

A second question is: **does our motivation affect the results?** Preliminary research suggests it does. Mice love to use the running wheel when it's put in their cages. They look like they enjoy using their body in this way. And the results in terms of neurogenesis are huge. But when mice are forced to exercise, as opposed to being allowed to run when they want to, the results appear to show that motivation influences neurogenesis. [16]

Here again we don't know the precise implications for humans, but it's probably not too big a jump to assume that for human beings, motivation is an even bigger factor in brain function than in mice. **Thus, it's better to find some form of exercise you enjoy and regularly do it, rather than forcing yourself to do something grudgingly because it's "good for you."** Since motivation counts for so much with people, and because humans don't tend to do things voluntarily that they don't enjoy, it's important to find forms of exercise where you revel in using your body.

So what if I don't like exercise and force myself to do it? **Your body and brain were designed by evolution to move about and exercise.** It's unnatural to sit in a chair or on the couch all day watching a computer screen or TV. But we get habituated to unnatural patterns like this, and then exercise becomes a grim duty rather than our joyful birthright. **The key to enjoying exercise is to allow yourself a long enough period of physical activity to unlearn the habit of sitting and allow your body's natural intelligence to awaken.**

Exercise takes practice. It's important to begin slowly and allow your body to build up strength and endurance. As you do so, your body changes and your brain changes along with it. Your body wakes up to the delight of moving and exercising its physical prowess. At some point things flip, and your body begins to feel so good when you exercise that it feels bad when you don't. Not exercising then makes you feel heavy, sluggish, dull. Exercise brings greater aliveness, which feels intrinsically good.

In learning not just to exercise but to awaken your body's natural enjoyment in exercising, it's necessary to keep going until it gets over this hump of resistance. Once you enjoy exercise and reclaim your body's intrinsic pleasure in moving, exercise is no longer a problem or a hard, heavy task you "should" do but something you take joy in doing. Then it becomes self-reinforcing in a virtuous cycle of feeling better and better.

The key is to find a form of exercise you enjoy. Forcing yourself to do something you just don't like soon backfires. Especially if you've been away from physical activity for a long time or are out of shape or overweight, then the very thought of exercise can seem daunting. **That's why it's crucial to find something you enjoy doing.** And certainly check with your physician to make sure you're physically fit enough to begin and what, if any, precautions to take.

The first choice for most people is walking. Getting out for a 20–30 minute walk three or four times a week will bring an aliveness into your life you didn't know was missing. Once you begin to appreciate walking, try walking a little faster and a little longer. Build up slowly, but get your lungs breathing faster as you feel ready for it. Slowly increase the time to 40–60 minutes.

In a *New York Times* interview (7/7/10) with neuroscience researcher Fred Gage, Ph.D., on this subject, he said, "even a fairly short period," of exercise "and a short distance seems to produce results." The key is to start moving.

Moving is enlivening. Our brains crave it. We just need to move through our initial resistance to discover our bodies' love of it. Then it becomes part of our lifestyle, something we do not only because it's good for us but because it feels so good.

Brain Healthy Running

It's well known that blows to the head slow neurogenesis, damage the connections between neurons, and increase the chances of getting Alzheimer's. That's why protecting your brain against sudden shocks to its delicate structures is a critical part of brain health.

Nobody knows just how much or how little roughness and physical shocks damage the delicate connections between neurons. Big shocks clearly do, like a concussion from a football game or a bike accident. A single concussion doubles a person's chances of developing Alzheimer's. Such shocks can cause permanent brain damage and even death. But smaller shocks also injure the brain.

This is an area where science is lagging. For a long time, it seemed fairly self-evident to even casual observers that the brutal jarring to the head that occurs in professional football was causing brain damage. The extraordinarily high rate of Alzheimer's disease in former NFL pros in their forties and fifties, the memory problems, the early deaths, these were all vigorously denied by the teams' owners and doctors. Then the science caught up with anecdotal reports and showed that indeed, professional football is extremely damaging to the brain. This resulted in a huge payout to the football players' association and more lawsuits continue.

It should be obvious that any exercise involving blows to the head is to be avoided. Boxing or martial arts that involve sparring and actual head blows are highly damaging to the brain and should be avoided.

How much jarring and shaking damages the brain's fragile connections and neural wiring? It's unknown. There are layers of protection for the brain, sheaths and liquid to cushion impacts of the delicate brain against the bony skull. But how much or how little impact is required? And to what degree is there individual variation on this, are some peoples' brains more vulnerable to injury than others'? This also is unknown.

Since we don't know what effects the mini-shocks from jogging have on brain function, we are best guided by common sense. It is clear that some forms of running are harder on the brain than others. Some runners come down with hard shocks on their heels and stiff legs so that it shakes their entire body (and brain). You can observe the shocks to the face and head with each stride. Other runners seem to glide like gazelles with a gentler step that cushions the upper body and brain. Given that we want to avoid any unnecessary roughness and protect the brain as much as possible, it is probably wise to run in the second way to reduce shocks to the brain.

One way to do this is to run so that the forefoot and toes touch the ground first rather than the classic "heel strike" that most people learned as children. This is the style of running recently popularized in the book *Born to Run,* which has a host of converts since its publication. "Chi running" is another approach to running in a low-impact way that emphasizes the mid-foot touching first instead of the hard landing of the heel strike. "Gentle running" and other popular approaches stress the importance of landing softly on the ground.

The easiest way to learn this is to run barefoot in a gym so that the outside ball of your foot and toes are the first to touch the floor. Then allow your legs to act as shock absorbers by bending at the knees to further cushion your stride. Keep your body fairly upright rather than leaning forward too much. (Chi running differs in this.) Allow your foot to glide softly onto the ground and then gently slide off the ground in one continuous motion, as your legs further absorb the impact. It takes a while to get used to it, so build up to it slowly and stop if pain comes. Once you learn it, this feels far less jarring than the old heel-strike method. Some people like to run barefoot, but this deprives us of another critical layer of cushioning. **Running shoes add important protection to both brain and foot.**

If you must do heel strikes, or if you're running downhill, the idea is to roll onto the backside of your heel and let your leg absorb the force. Glide across your heel as your weight shifts to the ball of your foot and toes, then gently roll off your foot. Try to imagine you're balancing a book on your head. Let your lower body absorb the impact so your head and brain can remain steady and just glide along without vibration. Here again, experiment to see what works for you. Run gently rather than with hard, unabsorbed shocks.

Low-impact running cushions the brain from the shocks and jolts that can shake the exceedingly delicate connections between neurons. Protecting this neural net from possible injury is a safeguard for brain health.

Brain healthy biking. It is probably obvious by now why biking with a helmet is recommended. The leading cause of permanent brain damage from athletics in the US is biking accidents, even more than football. This is because so many more people are biking than playing football at any given time.

Only half of cyclists wear a helmet regularly. Additionally, most of the helmets use obsolete technology that does not protect from the most frequent types of brain injury that occur in a biking accident. Current certification standards have not kept up with advancing science, which shows that "shear strain" on the brain due to rotational acceleration is the most common cause of concussions from bike accidents. Most helmets are designed for linear acceleration instead. Better to use a helmet that will protect your brain from the widest range of accidents instead of a helmet that is simply fashionable.

Biking accidents are the leading cause of preventable brain injury. And if you love mountain biking, be careful on the hard landings coming downhill and the sudden jolts that inevitably come. Use your legs and arms and upper body as shock absorbers.

* * * * * * * * *

Exercise is a powerful driver of neurogenesis, and nothing is as good as aerobic training. But to make the most of the newly born neurons exercise brings, other kinds of enrichment are needed to keep these neurons alive.

Touch

We tend to forget how important touch is in our lives. Mammals evolved with touch. As part of the mammalian brain, or limbic system, mammals as a species evolved to touch each other both emotionally and physically. Reptiles and fish don't have anything to do with their young after birth. Mammals lick, nestle, cuddle, wrestle, play with, hug, kiss, and touch their young and their mates and fellow creatures. **Touch stimulates neurogenesis.** [7,8]

Chimpanzees, our closest primate relatives, touch each other all the time, both when young and as adults. Chimps and other primates spend endless hours grooming each other, picking through each other's hair and body looking for lice, dirt, and giving each other a good massage and lots of stroking in the process. After chimps fight, they hug each other at the conclusion. When a whole tribe of monkeys experiences something intense, they all hug each other to calm and soothe and reestablish their bonds. **Touch expresses the social glue that holds them together, for whether human or non-human, all of us primates are social creatures.**

Human babies die if they aren't touched and held and caressed. When babies are orphaned or hospitalized, the nursing staff doesn't just feed them. They regularly need to pick them up, caress, touch, and stroke them, otherwise the babies die. **We are wired for touch.**

The mother instinctively picks up and holds her baby when it starts to cry. When the baby is distressed and cries, its immature nervous system hasn't yet learned to self-regulate. **When the mother picks up the baby to calm it, she allows her soothing touching and holding to regulate her baby's distressed nervous system.** The baby participates in the calmness of the mother's nervous system. The baby's immature nervous system synchronizes with the mother's nervous system, is regulated by it, and soon the baby is peaceful again. Over time the baby's nervous system gradually internalizes this repeated holding and learns to self-regulate.

But however good we are at self-regulation, both depth psychology and neuroscience agree that we continue to need others to help us regulate our emotions throughout our lifespans. Whether it's a reassuring touch on the shoulder by a friend or extended cuddling with a lover, touch helps us regulate our feelings. **Touching allows two nervous systems to synchronize and harmonize into a larger, more relaxed state in which both people feel better.**

There is a good deal of cultural variation in how much people touch. Cultures in warmer climates, native cultures especially, display lots of physical touching. Cultures in colder climates express less touch. Northern European and American cultures in particular display much less touching than many other cultures. Some Asian cultures engage in frequent touching while other Asian cultures show considerably less.

America is a touch-starved culture. One study showed 75% of Americans want more hugs and touch while one third receive no touch at all in their lives. Although our primate instincts cry out for touch, it is prohibited in most circles, partly out of fear of being sexual and partly out of pure repression. **Yet our bodies and brains hunger for touch.**

Touch stimulates the release of oxytocin, the so-called love hormone which helps bonding and attachment. Oxytocin is secreted during childbirth, nursing, sex, and orgasm. Touch and hugging also stimulate the release of oxytocin. **Oxytocin reduces stress hormones such as cortisol, lowers blood pressure, increases heart health, boosts immunity, lessens depression, eases fatigue, and increases neurogenesis.** [23]

A 20 second hug followed by 10 minutes of holding hands has a strong anti-stress response that lowers blood pressure and heart rate. Even a 10 second hug each day leads to hormonal and bodily changes that improve health.

Touch increases neurogenesis. The more children are touched growing up, the higher their rate of adult neurogenesis. The more adults are touched, the higher their rate of neurogenesis. Touch is good for us (provided it's not unwanted or inappropriate). The key is trust. If we trust the person touching or hugging us, oxytocin is released, then we feel relaxed and calmed. But if we don't know or trust the person or if the touch is unwanted, we feel more stress, not less. **Trust is key.** If we know and trust the person and welcome their touch, it's good for our brains and unleashes a cascade of health benefits.

In the 1940s and '50s a researcher named Harry Harlow experimented with raising monkeys and giving them a choice between two inanimate mothers: a wire mother and a terry-cloth mother, each with a picture of a monkey for a face. The monkeys overwhelmingly preferred the terry-cloth mother, even when it was the wire mother who had the bottle for feeding. They would go to the wire mother when hungry, but immediately after eating they would rush back to the terry-cloth mother, which they would also cling to whenever frightened or alarmed.

Of course even though the terry-cloth mother was cuddlier, it couldn't touch back and provide the social interaction necessary for development. It will come as no surprise that both groups were very maladjusted and never really recovered, but **those with the wire mother only were much more disturbed, anxious, and depressed, with a lifetime of lowered immunity.** Those with the touchable terry-cloth mothers fared much better. We know now that monkeys with no real mothers have lifelong levels of elevated stress hormones and anxiety.

As technology progresses and people spend more time with smart phones, computers, and tablets than with other human beings, we are creating a generation raised by wire mothers, kids whose social interaction is mediated through technology and are less and less comfortable with direct human contact. One of the most wrenching sights in modern life is a crying baby in a stroller reaching out to its mother while the oblivious mother is busy on her cell phone, texting or playing a game.

While cell phones and texting allow for a greater sense of ongoing connection in one way, they are still a reduced form of connection, a virtual connection. As virtual connections replace actually seeing and hearing and touching the physical presence of who we're talking to, some part of our nervous system contracts and feels starved. Actual contact becomes scarier rather than more nourishing. Texting is no substitute for touching. Whenever possible, call someone rather than text, or better yet be with someone in real life.

As increasing numbers live alone in our society, we are a more and more touch-starved culture. **When we aren't touched parts of our bodies and brains go numb.** This is an immense tragedy, no less so because it's easy to become inured to the pain around it. What can be done?

The first step is knowing our needs. If I don't know what my needs are, I can't meet them very well. Once I know, I can better meet them. If you live alone, try initiating touch with friends or those you can trust. Consider getting massages regularly. There are now proven benefits from having a pet, such as increased oxytocin released from petting and holding a dog or cat, so consider this as well. If you have kids, make sure to touch them and hug them often, not just for their sake but for yours.

Many couples become estranged and touch very little if ever. Something dies in a relationship when this happens. It is generally a sign something needs serious attention in the relationship, and couples therapy is worth exploring. **If you're in a relationship, touch often.** Your brain and your partner's brain will appreciate it.

Take time away from whatever your electronic wire monkey is to be with and touch other flesh and blood people. Every brain will benefit, the one who touches and the one who receives the touch.

Sexual Experience

Now here's a good reason to have sex: it increases neurogenesis. To find out that sex is not only a good form of moderate exercise but actually increases neurogenesis has to be one of the best and most useful discoveries of science over the last decade. Sex restores the middle-age decline in neurogenesis to youthful levels. [2, 24, 26]

This discovery is hardly surprising. **Most people intuitively sense that sex is intrinsically healthy and life affirming.** It is important to note, however, that for the effects to last, sex must be ongoing. One or two sexual experiences aren't enough to sustain the effect on neurogenesis.

Not only does sexual experience increase neurogenesis, it also:

- improves immunity
- cuts the risk of heart attack in half in men who have sex twice a week or more
- reduces stress
- improves sleep
- lowers blood pressure

Further, the hormone oxytocin is released during sex and orgasm. This enhances bonding and loving attachment, which has physical and emotional benefits. [19, 23]

Knowing that sex stimulates neurogenesis is only part of the story. The next question is: what kind of sex? That is, sex under what kinds of conditions? Here we again run into the limitations of experiments with non-human mammals. Yes, you put a mouse in an environment without sex or with sex, and neurogenesis increases when the mouse has sex. But people have a much more complicated relationship to sex than mice.

It makes sense that just good, physical sex between two consenting adults who enjoy each other's body would provide the kind of brain stimulation that increases neurogenesis, just like it does for mice. Many men and increasing numbers of women report being able to enjoy good physical sex in this way. So far, so good.

However, in human beings sex is tied to emotional experience in a far more complex way than it is for other mammals. The studies on the effects of touch are relevant here. For touch to be helpful for reducing stress, it needs to be welcomed and from someone we trust. Otherwise it adds to our stress. (It should go without saying that traumatic sex such as rape or abuse falls under the category of extreme stress that almost brings neurogenesis to a halt rather than falling under the category of sex. That's not what we're talking about here. Rather we are considering the everyday, consensual sexual experience of most people.) **For many women and increasing numbers of men (especially as they mature) sex is intimately bound up with the emotional connection to the other person.**

Having sex under pressured circumstances or with unresolved resentment in the air is much different than the lovemaking between two soul mates madly in love with each other. Current research suggests that the first situation may result in more stress, anger, and other feelings that work against neurogenesis, while the second situation may result in even greater neurogenesis than straightforward physical sex. For most people, emotion trumps the act when it comes to sexual experience.

Sleep

Recent research shows that most of us badly minimize how important sleep is. Sleep is our most restorative activity. After a good night's sleep we wake up refreshed, renewed, ready for a new day. Our bodies and brains repair and renew themselves during sleep. It seems intuitively obvious that sleep would increase neurogenesis, and science confirms that indeed, it does. [9,10]

Most neurogenesis occurs during sleep. Sleep stimulates neurogenesis. There's a catch though. **We need a full night's sleep, meaning about 7–8 hours each night.** Less than this and neurogenesis declines.

Many people in developed countries don't get nearly enough sleep. Most Americans report getting only 6.5 hours of sleep on weeknights. According to the National Sleep Foundation (NSF) only 4 out of 10 people report getting a good night's sleep every night or almost every night of the week. One third of Americans report getting less sleep than they need to function well. Between 50 and 70 million Americans have a diagnosable chronic sleep disorder.

Even a single night of 4–6 hours of sleep reduces cognitive function the next day. It reduces your ability to integrate or put facts together and impedes your ability to pay attention to your environment. Four percent of all fatal car crashes are due to sleepiness. Figures from the National Highway Traffic Safety Administration (NTSB) estimate sleepy drivers cause 1,550 deaths, 71,000 injuries, and more than 100,000 accidents each year.

Not getting enough sleep is now seen as a major health hazard. Not sleeping enough, or having disrupted sleep due to shift work, has been identified as a carcinogen and is linked to:

- weight gain (because hormones are thrown out of balance. People deprived of sleep eat about 300 extra calories a day, which quickly adds up over time)
- cancer (tumor growth is accelerated two or three times in lab animals with severe sleep disruption)
- heart and cardiovascular disease, including stroke
- high blood pressure
- depression
- elevated blood glucose levels and higher risk of diabetes
- increased risk of an auto accident
- lowered immune function for all diseases
- altered gene expression

Sleep is an essential part of brain and overall body health, and its true importance is only now being understood. [31]

Hundreds of millions of years of evolutionary development have geared humans and other creatures to the cycle of day and

night. Evolution adapted our bodies' circadian rhythms to light and dark—the rising and setting of the sun. But when electricity was discovered just a hundred years ago, a blink of the eye in evolutionary time, our internal clock was suddenly thrown off-kilter.

Suddenly human beings could determine how much light or dark they wanted. It is believed that sleep went from ten hours a night to seven or eight as electric lighting became widespread. Just in the last 10 years it's estimated that Americans sleep 38 minutes less per night on weekends. But seven or eight hours may be the physical limit to how little sleep we can get and still stay healthy. **Less than seven or eight hours of sleep wreaks havoc with our immune system and brain.**

Staying up late with bright lights, TVs, computer screens—all this is brand-new to the human brain. Jangled nervous systems, hormonal balances out of whack, immune system dysfunctions, and disrupted sleep patterns are the result.

So many of the body's repair systems work during sleep.

- Muscles that were broken down during the day are built back up.
- Organs are repaired.
- Memory consolidation occurs.
- The immune system is strengthened.
- The brain cleans itself by removing waste and toxins.
- Neurogenesis is heightened.

Research published in a fall 2013 issue of *Science* 18 shows that the brain has its own newly discovered cleaning system for removing the toxic waste that builds up during the day. Just as the lymphatic system eliminates cellular waste products from the body, the brain has its own system that is sealed off from the rest of the body by the blood-brain barrier.

Called the "glymphatic system" in deference to the glial cells that organize this process, the glymphatic system flushes waste from the brain back into the circulatory system, where the liver eventually eliminates it. This process also flushes out much more of the beta-amyloid, which is implicated in Alzheimer's disease, than develops during the day.

Think of a fish tank. Without a filter to clean the water, the fish soon die in that closed system due to the buildup of toxic waste. Up until now it was a mystery how the brain cleaned out its waste and toxic buildup, since it too is a closed system. **The discovery of the glymphatic system revealed that the brain has a highly sophisticated cleaning and filtering system at work.**

The fluid-filled area between neurons is called interstitial space, and while awake it makes up about 20% of the brain's volume. But during sleep it appears to swell by 30% as cerebrospinal fluid flushes the brain of toxic waste, much like a bath or shower for the brain. This system works in mice, goats, dogs, baboons, and, it is assumed, humans, because a bigger brain makes such a cleaning system even more important.

This research shows why sleep is so important to brain health and body health. **When brain waste and toxins build up due to lack of sleep, we think less well, memory is disrupted, stress hormones aren't cleared, immunity is lowered, anxiety and depression increase, and neurogenesis is slowed.** Washing out the toxic residue from a day of wakefulness keeps the brain clean and fresh. When toxic residues accumulate, the short-term result is a foggy brain. The long-term result may be an increase in Alzheimer's, Parkinson's, and other neurodegenerative diseases. The clearance of beta-amyloids and tau is drastically reduced when we sleep less.

The stress of modern life keeps the adrenaline pumping so much we hardly even feel like we need sleep. But higher levels of stress hormones alone will reduce neurogenesis, as we've already learned. **Not sleeping adds to this effect by keeping higher levels of stress hormones in circulation.** [18]

Once the stress hormones are surging, it becomes difficult to fall asleep even though you're exhausted. After a while you get used to running on less sleep, and caffeine and sugar can keep you going temporarily during the day, although this short-term solution only makes the long-term situation worse.

A single night or two of poor sleep doesn't seem to slow down neurogenesis. Rather it's a pattern of disrupted or not enough sleep that causes neurogenesis to decline.

The majority of people need seven or eight hours a night. Individual variation, however, shows that six and nine hours are the upper and lower limits, respectively, for most everyone. **You have to see what you need.** If you're tired during the day, find yourself yawning or wanting naps, you probably need more sleep.

Quantity is important but so is the quality of sleep for neurogenesis. We need to sleep in a dark environment. Sleeping with light in your room decreases neurogenesis and impairs cognitive performance. [17] If you must have lights, such as from a nightlight or clock, better to have red, orange, or amber light than the blue wavelengths of the spectrum, which have a more disruptive effect on circadian rhythms and melatonin production. Many people report disrupted sleep due to EMF exposure, so keep cell phones, Wi-Fi, electrical devices, and alarm clocks away from your head and body while you sleep.

Melatonin is a hormone secreted by the pineal gland at night during sleep. **Besides increasing neurogenesis and immunity, melatonin has antioxidant and anti-inflammatory properties, and it regulates our circadian rhythms.** [11, 28, 29] Melatonin production declines with age, and correspondingly, sleep disturbances increase with age. To offset declining melatonin production many people use a melatonin supplement to slow the effects of aging and as a sleep aid that doesn't have the hangover of sleeping pills when taken in the right dose (anywhere from 1–30 mg).

Good sleep hygiene includes:

- Developing a routine around sleep that trains your body to fall asleep at a regular time.
- Avoid stimulating movies, TV, reading an hour before bed. Also put your work away to help reduce stress and feel calmer before sleep.
- Unplug from your computer screen 30–60 minutes before sleeping and lower the lights. Bright lights impede melatonin production and sleepiness.
- Avoid fluids, grains, and sugars before sleep, as these raise your blood sugar and postpone sleep or cause you to get up to urinate.
- Avoid caffeine in the afternoon. Some people clear caffeine very slowly and need to stop in the morning; others are more tolerant and can ingest later. Best to stop entirely if falling asleep is a problem.
- Avoid alcohol before sleep. Its initial impact is drowsiness, but this is counteracted by awakening several hours later and preventing the deeper stages of sleep from occurring, which is when most healing of the body happens.

- Reduce stress in your life. Better than any sleep aid is finding what stresses are disturbing your sleep and reducing or eliminating them.

Only now are we beginning to understand just how important sleep is to health and rejuvenation. The brain literally renews itself during sleep via neurogenesis and deep cleansing. Making a good night's sleep a priority can change your life in more ways than you realize.

Doing New Things, Being in Novel Environments, New Sensory Stimulation

Our brains thrive on new stimulation. Novel, ever-changing environments engage the brain and stimulate neurogenesis. But it's a matter of degrees. Too much new stimulation can be overwhelming and stressful, which impairs neurogenesis. On the other hand, too little new stimulation, as in a deprived environment, also reduces neurogenesis. It's another Goldilocks dilemma: **we need just the right balance between new stimulation and safe and familiar stimulation.**

Finding the "sweet spot" between the monotony of a boring, deprived environment and the overstimulation of an overwhelming dazzle of lights and colors is a very individual matter. Some people have a high need and tolerance for intense sensory displays and find such environments exciting and engaging. Other people have a more sensitive nervous system that thrives on subtle cues and hues. There is no "one size fits all" here.

In between monotony and overstimulation is optimal engagement. It's this optimal engagement we're looking to create in our lives. Going to either extreme slows down neurogenesis.

Finding the "Middle Way" of optimal engagement enhances neurogenesis and promotes the survival of new neurons.

In mice this means providing new places to explore in their cages, new tunnels, nesting materials, and running wheels on a daily basis. In other words, variations on the theme of a relatively stable environment that presents new, ever-changing sensory cues, places to explore and engage.

This translates into many different things for people. Travel, for example, is one way of producing novel, ever-changing environments to explore in a context of relative safety and stability, providing one has the resources to so do. (However, traveling without enough money or in dangerous areas or war zones can be scary, stressful, and even traumatic, all of which interferes with neurogenesis.) Ordinary travel and tourism is a way to see new sights, meet new people, try new foods and smells, hear new sounds, and discover different cultures. **Travel expands our worlds and our brains.**

We don't need to travel to a foreign country to experience this. All that's required is going to a new part of your state or city or region, exploring some part of your local environment that is off the beaten track—at least *your* beaten track. Breaking up your routine to try new things is key.

This can also mean having new colors in your home and on your walls. It's not that you redecorate every day, but that you provide yourself with sensory stimulation, colors, and sights that increase the complexity of your space, ways for your eyes to engage.

It means meeting new people. (More on this later.) It means trying new activities. It means making an effort to enlarge your world and overcoming the entropic tendency to settle down into a lifeless, stale routine.

It means exposing yourself to new movies, TV shows, and other entertainment. Here again science has not yet defined the limits, but it seems reasonable that watching movies or TV is more stimulating than staring at a blank wall for days and nights on end. But just watching TV and movies is no substitute for going out into the world and living.

Here again it's a question of context and balance. Watching TV and movies is a passive activity that does engage the brain at one level, but at other levels it leaves us passively receptive. **In fact too many hours watching TV correlates with lower cognitive function.** [25] Watching soap operas is no substitute for a life, on the one hand. But it may be better than solitary confinement, on the other. You need to find the right balance *for you*.

Trying out new cultural activities is another dimension of this. Going to concerts, museums, plays, lectures, community meetings, and cultural gatherings of all kinds enlarges your world, opens you to something new, enriches your life, and provides the kind of stimulation that increases neurogenesis.

The human mind has a tendency to follow routine. This makes for efficiency, so the brain doesn't have to work hard to figure everything out for the first time. But carried to the extreme it results in a dull, monotonous life with few surprises. We all need novelty for highest brain function. You just need to find what is right for your unique nature.

Music Is Good and Silence Is Golden

It was music to my ears when I first read research showing music can increase neurogenesis. [12, 13] General noise pollution, as would be expected, decreases neurogenesis, probably because it is stressful. But music increases neurogenesis both in babies in utero as well as adults.

Mice respond well to music, at least to Mozart and other classical music used in the experiments. For people it probably depends on the type of music you like and how loud it is. If you can't stand heavy metal rock at loud volumes, listening to that kind of music will probably not increase neurogenesis and may well decrease it, just as any loud, stressful noise would. But if you love this kind of music at high volume, such a musical diet may well be perfect for you. (Just be careful of how many decibels you expose your ears to.)

Natural sounds also promote relaxation and recovery from stress. Sounds such as birds singing, crickets chirping, a stream bubbling, wind blowing the leaves of a tree, and the waves of the ocean have a soothing, calming effect on people. [14]

Construction noises, cars, trucks, leaf blowers, and other sounds of civilization raise stress levels and reduce neurogenesis. These sounds produce a small but measurable increase in stress that is all the more insidious because we don't usually notice it. It becomes "background." But this background noise takes a toll on our health. A recent study showed that living near an airport increased risk of cardiovascular disease by 3.5%. Not huge, but who needs any higher risk level? [15]

What is most surprising is that silence increases neurogenesis more than music. Silence may promote a kind of alert awareness that enhances brain function and stimulates neurogenesis. While it can be difficult to find or create silence in an urban setting, it's clear that silence helps brain health.

Nature

Nature is good for your brain. This should come as no surprise since the human brain has developed over a few hundred million years of evolution to be perfectly adapted to the natural world. Of course our brains thrive in nature.

It should also come as no surprise that cities and human-made environments of concrete and traffic and pollution and artificial lights are not healthy for the brain. They create stresses that decrease neurogenesis.

Research shows that natural environments stimulate neurogenesis more than artificial ones. When mice or monkeys are allowed to live in natural settings, the increase in their rate of neurogenesis outstrips what happens in captivity. [14]

There is so much more complexity to nature than a cage or room that it makes sense such complexity of stimulation is better for neurogenesis than painted walls or cages. **This has important implications for people because we all live in artificial environments.** Anyone who lives in a house or apartment lives in an artificially constructed environment—a cage for humans, if you will.

By now there is a great deal of evidence to show the brain benefits of nature and the harmful effects of being deprived of nature. Eco-psychology has shown how healing nature can be for anxiety, depression, ADD, and ADHD, as well as a host of other symptoms. There are demonstrated cognitive and emotional benefits to walking 50 minutes in a pine forest vs. a walk through city streets. **Walking in nature reduces stress hormones and increases DHEA, the "youth hormone" that stimulates neurogenesis but which declines with stress and age.** [14]

Being in nature is a total sensory immersion. Breaking this experience down into its component parts reveals that each sense is stimulated by nature. The sounds of nature are relaxing and soothing. Nature is visually complex and rich. It also provides the full spectrum of light waves so important for mood. Office workers in the interior of buildings show higher rates of depression and stress than those who have windows to the outside. Getting full spectrum lighting with more of the blue part of the spectrum that most indoor lighting leaves out is helpful although slightly more expensive.

We know that one type of depression, seasonal affective depression or SAD, is caused by inadequate amounts of sunlight or full spectrum light. Light therapy has been shown to help people feel better and recover from SAD. Since depression involves reduced neurogenesis, it is hard to avoid the strong possibility that reduced lighting reduces neurogenesis. While the definitive study has not yet been done, it would not be hard to show if this is indeed the case.

Students who have outside views, either in their college dorms or in their elementary school classrooms and cafeterias, do better on standardized academic tests. Even having more trees and shrubs along highways reduces road rage, anger, and impulsivity in drivers. [14] Indoor plants reduce eyestrain, boost creativity, and increase attention span in workers.

Try to spend time in nature or a park. Even if it's just a matter of getting outside and walking around to look at the sky and clouds, make an effort to experience the natural world. Even better is living closer to nature or taking frequent trips to nature. Exercise in nature if possible. Research shows people exercise longer and better in nature than in a gym.

Bringing nature into your home is another way to come closer to the natural world. Plants and flowers bring living energy, natural smells, and complexity into your space. **Find spaces that have windows to nature whenever possible.** Windows that look out on concrete and brick are not nearly as good, but they are better than no windows at all.

Future Dreams

In the future, nature, plants, and flowers will be part of every building. Architects will design with nature in mind, and the cold, sterile, soulless buildings of the past will be replaced by visually interesting, colorful inner spaces that always look out onto some natural setting.

No one will sit for eight hours a day anymore. Getting up at regular intervals and moving around will be part of all healthy workplaces.

Exercise is built into every job so that workers' morale will be high. In the same way that taxes and social security benefits are part of every job now, so will a variety of aerobic exercise options be a part of all work situations in the future. Exercise will simply be an enjoyable part of everyday life, like eating or getting dressed each day, and the health of the citizenry will be better than it has ever been.

Cultural inhibitions around touch will have faded away in the late 21st century after child abuse and sexual violence in all forms ended, so friends and family will allow themselves to freely express caring touch without fear.

Summary

As you can see, there are many things we can do to stimulate neurogenesis at the level of the body. One theme of this book is that neurogenesis is a lifestyle. The more ways we stimulate our brain, the more robust the effect on enhancing our life and on neurogenesis. Aerobic exercise, touch, sex, sensory novelty, music, and nature all stimulate neurogenesis.

CHAPTER 5

HEART

Home is where the heart is.

By now it's clear that an enriched environment both stimulates neurogenesis and keeps the new neurons alive. [34, 42]

A main ingredient of an enriched environment is emotional stimulation. However, this stimulation needs to be the *right kind*.

The right kind of emotional stimulation leads to increased neurogenesis as well as emotional fulfillment. The wrong kind is neurotoxic and disrupts neurogenesis, even kills brain cells.

Emotion Organizes the Brain

We tend to be unaware of how we spend our lives swimming in a sea of emotion. Neuroscience emphasizes how essential emotion is in organizing the brain and how key relationships are in this process.

Most people take their everyday relationships for granted, so much so that they tend to fade into the background like wallpaper.

Yet these everyday relationships and how you feel throughout the day exert an immense effect upon your brain and neurogenesis.

The brain is designed for joy, love, interest, and excitement. It thrives in positive emotional conditions. Neurogenesis is ignited when you feel good. The brain functions at peak capacity when you feel your best.

The brain shrivels in the opposite conditions of stress, despair, lack of engagement, and depression. Neurogenesis and BDNF levels drop markedly. When you feel bad, and your brain functions poorly.

Optimal Emotional Stimulation Increases Neurogenesis

In general, optimal emotional stimulation means feeling good rather than bad most of the time. Of course, everyone wants to be happy. But it's much more than this. **Optimal emotional stimulation involves positive emotional engagement with our lives, our work, and our relationships.**

The result is a zone of emotional fulfillment: happiness, love, joy, gratitude, openness, and interest. This zone is the goal of life and key to promoting neurogenesis. Of course no one lives exclusively in this zone, and negative feelings are inevitable. But living well means living in these positive emotional states most of the time.

Affirmative, life-enhancing relationships that allow us to feel a deep, loving connection with others go hand in hand with feeling good. These kinds of relationships both bring about and are a hallmark of fulfillment and well-being. **Caring, warm relationships like these are neuroprotective and enhance both neurogenesis and our immune systems.** [6, 11, 18]

The second zone consists of their opposites—stress, anxiety, fear, depression, anger, isolation and loneliness—as chronic states.

These opposites reduce neurogenesis and open the door to illness by undermining our immune systems. [6, 20, 24]

Negative relationships often accompany these negative emotional states. Relationships that are stressful, upsetting, chronically angry, fear inducing, or domineering reduce neurogenesis, seriously risk our physical health, and can bring about disorders linked to such depression, anxiety, or trauma. Even the lack of relationships—social isolation that results in loneliness—reduces neurogenesis and is a bigger risk factor for heart disease and depression than smoking, diet, or other lifestyle factors. [18, 21]

Chronic negative emotional states and negative relationships decrease neurogenesis and shrink the hippocampus.

The first zone of positive feelings increases neurogenesis while the second zone of negative feelings decreases neurogenesis. While this seems to make such intuitive sense that it's like a blinding flash of the obvious, living primarily in the first zone is much easier said than done. What exactly does a zone of positive feelings mean in terms of daily living?

David

David had a tough childhood. Bullied by his three older brothers, an angry father, and an overwhelmed and not very protective mother, he entered therapy hoping to find a relationship. "Every time I get together with a girl," he explained, "It ends within a year. Why am I so unlucky in love?"

David had some friends from his work as a paramedic, but he kept other men at a distance. He'd learned early on he couldn't trust men after his brothers bullied him without mercy for so many years. In his work he put up with an abusive boss who seemed to single him out to pick on, but he didn't complain because he just figured that's how men in authority are.

What closeness he had in life was with a younger sister and occasional girlfriends while their relationship lasted. He was scared of relationships and even more scared of real intimacy and vulnerability, so he kept even women he thought were safe at an emotional distance. He battled PTSD around relationships that left him isolated, anxious, and longing for connection. He had health issues that may have been exacerbated by a reduced immune system caused by his continual state of stress. In his early forties, he also worried his memory was going downhill.

Our work touched on all parts of his life. Physically he worked out, but his diet was high in carbs and sugar, which he was open to changing. Mentally he was able to challenge his beliefs that all men were out to get him. Spiritually we experimented with meditation practices to bring a sense of peace to his mind and body. It was on the emotional level that we focused most of our attention, on working through his PTSD around being bullied and his fears about relationships.

Over the course of a couple years, he began to engage more deeply with others, letting more men into his life and opening up to a new girlfriend with whom he felt safe. As he felt less stressed in his relationships, he was able to transfer to another part of the city with a boss whom he genuinely liked. His anxiety decreased dramatically. His mood brightened.

"I had no idea I was so scared. I now see I was too scared to admit how scared I was. Fear distorts everything! It feels so good to be able to relax and to start enjoying being with people."

Translating Animal Data into Human Terms

In this section we come to the problem of applying the data from animal research to human beings. As stated earlier, since humans share the basic brain structures and neurotransmitters with other mammals, much of this research is directly applicable. At the level of the body and physical things (like exercise and diet) it is a relatively easy jump to humans (although even here future research may show that a particular nutrient has different effects).

The level of the heart and emotional experience involves a little more translation, for even though mice and monkeys share basic emotional states with us, humans' emotional lives are more varied and complex. Four experiments will illustrate how applicable this animal research data is for people and neurogenesis—see just how easy it is to put yourself into the position of a mouse or monkey.

Experiment #1: When you put a mouse together with other friendly mice it can play with, mate with, explore, and run around with, neurogenesis shoots up dramatically. The positive feelings that this generates go along with higher immune function, lower blood pressure, reduced heart disease, and other positive biomarkers of health.

For mice a key part of an "enriched environment" is other mice. **But just any other mice won't do—they must be nice mice.**

Experiment #2: When you take one of these same mice and put it in a cage with a big bully mouse that beats it up (pins it down, bites it, behaves in a dominant, aggressive way), this mouse experiences stress. When you then make this mouse live next to the big bully mouse, this stress becomes chronic, and very shortly the intense anxiety makes the mouse give up and become depressed. This is known as the "social defeat" model of depression, and it slows neurogenesis to a crawl.

Along with much reduced neurogenesis, blood pressure increases and the risk of heart disease goes up, while immune function and other biomarkers of health go down very quickly. The mouse looks just like a human who's depressed would. It is lethargic, displays anhedonia (less pleasure seeking), lowered testosterone, and reduced sexual and exploratory behavior. Mouse depression looks remarkably like human depression. And depression—whether in mice, monkeys, or humans—means impaired neurogenesis.

Here are two other experiments that come at this from a different angle.

Experiment #3: Give a solitary male monkey a mild shock and he experiences stress. Glucocorticoids and other stress hormones pour into his system, blood pressure goes up, and immunity goes down along with neurogenesis. But give this monkey one or two other monkeys from his troop and everything changes. Being in the company of friends while getting a shock relaxes him, stress levels and blood pressure drop quickly. The social support from his friends boosts his emotional resilience. He is "protected" from stress and rebounds quickly from the shock.

Experiment #4: But then, instead of being with his friends, put him with a monkey from another troop, a stranger. His stress levels soar. They go higher than if he was alone. He becomes more anxious, blood pressure increases, neurogenesis slackens.

Good relationships are neuroprotective, they reduce stress and depression while increasing neurogenesis. Bad relationships create stress and depression and decrease neurogenesis.

This is the paradox of relationships. We need them for love and support, to reduce stress and feel good. **Good relationships give us the emotional stimulation that makes us feel good— loved, reassured, joyful, interested—and stimulate neurogenesis.**

But relationships can also be a major source of stress and make us feel terrible. **Bad relationships make us stressed out, anxious, hurt, angry, unloved, depressed, and slow down neurogenesis.**

Additionally, good quality relationships are essential to feeling good, and emotions are our key to finding and cultivating good relationships. Our emotional brains are our guidance mechanisms for navigating our interpersonal worlds.

Feeling good requires skillful navigation of our emotions. Becoming skilled takes time as we learn to listen to our hearts' guidances. This means knowing what feelings to act on and what feelings *not* to act on, what feelings to be guided by and what feelings to overcome. It means knowing how to relate to our feelings.

Understanding the Emotional Brain

Our emotional brains are integrated with our other two brains, the reptilian physical brain that manages our body and the neocortex responsible for higher thinking. But our emotional brains run much more of the show than we'd like to admit. Far from being coolly rational, logical, or dispassionate, we are governed by our feelings much more than we acknowledge.

Depth psychology from Freud on has emphasized how central emotion is to the psyche. Neuroscience is now confirming this. Humans share an emotional brain, or limbic system, with mice and monkeys and all other mammals. Granted, our emotional lives are more complex and differentiated, just as our ability to regulate our emotional states is far more developed. But emotion guides and motivates us throughout our days. **Emotion is central to how the entire brain is organized.**

According to neuroscientist Daniel Siegel, M.D., emotion wires the brain and organizes how we experience the world. Emotion shapes how information and energy flow across brain systems and integrate the various data streams—sensations, thoughts, memories, desires, planning, perception—into an integrated experience of living. [1]

How we feel colors our whole lives. It affects everything we do. It even affects our health and immune systems. The field of psychoneuroimmunology investigates how the psyche and brain affect the immune system, and it has shown over the past two decades how negative emotion and split-off emotion seriously impair our immunity. [2] Optimists live longer than pessimists (presumably because expecting the worst results in a kind of constant, low-grade stress that erodes the body's defenses). [20, 21, 44]

Emotion organizes our experience of the world in several different ways:

- As *information*. Emotions give us information about the world that we just can't get any other way. No matter how much we think about a situation, thought can only tell us so much. Logic alone spins off into infinite possibilities. Feelings are needed to tell us who to trust or what data are most essential.

- As *a method of evaluation*. Emotion assesses people and situations. At the simplest level, feelings let us know if something is good or bad, whether we want more or less. Feelings are the guidance mechanism for the interpersonal world we live in.

- As *a form of communication*. We are constantly receiving and interpreting the emotional states of those around us, just as we in turn are signaling our feelings to others. The right brain understands what others are feeling immediately and nonverbally, through facial expression, tone of voice, body language, and other cues. We are always scanning our environment for emotional signals. [4, 33]

- As *motivation*. Everything we do or say has a feeling behind it. To do something implies some motivation for doing it. Whether we're aware of it or not (and often we aren't) every voluntary action in our lives is motivated by some feeling. Otherwise we wouldn't do it.

- As *a direction for action*. Emotion guides how we act. Implicit in our feelings is a sense of the next step forward. When we don't know how we feel, we don't know what to do.

- As *meaning*. Emotion lets us know in what ways events are significant to us. Although meaning also has a cognitive component, it's the emotional dimension that gives the felt experience of meaning. The same neural circuits that process meaning also process feeling.

- As *an integrating function*. Emotion brings together the different strands of our experiences—thinking, sensing, feeling, imagining—into a coherent whole so we can make sense of the world and live highly complex lives.

The Wisdom of Emotion

We live in a sea of emotion, and the heart's guidance shapes our lives. Pervasive, like water for a fish, currents of emotion invisibly steer us this way and that, draw us toward some people and away from others, drive us into some situations and repel us from others.

Emotion is an appraisal process that lets us know, at the simplest level, whether something is good or bad, nourishing or

toxic. Emotion has a valance: positive or negative. At times our feeling states coalesce into discrete emotions such as anger, shame, or fear. At other times our emotional states are less defined and experienced more as a current of feeling, either positive or negative. But however defined or vague, our feelings tell us about our present states and our environments throughout the day. [3]

Only by understanding and following our feelings do we find positive relationships and steer clear of negative ones. When we feel joyous, loving, prized, and appreciated, we are probably in a relationship that is emotionally nourishing and brain healthy. If we feel persistently bad in a relationship, it's important to ask if that relationship is worth continuing if it can't be transformed.

Feeling Good Is Linked to Good Relationships

There is a close connection in human beings between feeling good and the quality of our relationships. Satisfying time with friends, a lover, work colleagues, a teacher or mentor produces an emotional state of well-being: warm feelings of connection, caring or love, appreciation, admiration, enjoyment.

We can feel good on our own, for example, enjoying nature or music. But soon we long for other people; we want to share it or communicate our experiences. Sometimes it's possible to feel good from having done something well, such as completed a job, created a work of art, or reached a personal goal. But even this is usually connected to the hope that others will recognize us or we can join with others in our enjoyment.

As depth psychology has learned, our emotional states depend upon the states of our interpersonal worlds. Do we have people in our lives who truly see and love our real selves, or are we trying to get love for a self-image we've been carrying around since childhood? Do we have friends we can relax around? Are we connected to a teacher or mentor who helps guide us in our jobs or lives? Can we be deeply intimate, loving, and vulnerable with a significant other or with close friends?

This is a realm that psychotherapy has studied for decades. Therapy has become increasingly effective in showing people how to move away from negative states and relationships and toward positive states and relationships.

Love Increases Neurogenesis

Love in all its forms—romantic love, making love (sexual experiences), loving relationships with family, pets, and friendships—increases neurogenesis by increasing the hormone oxytocin and by other mechanisms not yet well understood. [9, 12]

We all need love. Throughout our lives—from the time we're born till our last breath—to love and to be loved is our core need. When we don't get love or give love, something inside shrivels up. **It also appears that without love our brains shrivel up as well.**

Oxytocin increases trust, empathy, and other feelings of closeness. Oxytocin is known as the "love hormone" because it's released during loving experiences such as:

- immediately after childbirth and during nursing
- sex
- orgasm
- bonding and attachment experiences
- parenting
- close relationships, deep sharing
- emotional intimacy

Since the emotional brain of mice and monkeys and other mammals so closely resembles that of humans, we'd expect that oxytocin would be involved in bonding experiences with other mammals. And indeed it is.

The prairie vole mates for life in a monogamous relationship. Prairie voles also have the highest amount of oxytocin of all vole species. Voles with little oxytocin are not monogamous, nor do they form pair bonds for life.

When men and women kiss or hug, oxytocin levels soar. Oxytocin even works between species. After someone pets a dog for five minutes, oxytocin levels rise in both the person and the dog. **Oxytocin stimulates neurogenesis.** [32]

In most modern cultures people look for fulfillment in a romantic relationship. The depths of love and intimate connection we experience in a close sexual relationship far surpass what most casual relationships offer. Whether we're lucky enough to find our "soul mate" or whether we but briefly feel such love, our lives are forever altered by this experience.

As the previous chapter touched on, sexual behavior seems to be more connected to emotion in humans than other animals. However, even mice show sensitivity to emotional dynamics that influence neurogenesis.

Sexual and romantic interactions influence brain plasticity as well as neurogenesis. A single 30-minute episode of male-female interaction increased neurogenesis in one species of rats. Female mice showed increases in neurogenesis simply from being around a male mouse for a short period each day for two weeks. However, most studies with other mammals indicate that ongoing sexual experience is necessary for neurogenesis to occur. [15]

Sexual hormones play a role in neurogenesis as well. Being around potential mates increases testosterone in males, and higher estrogen levels in females leads to greater sexual interest. [34-36] Estrogen and testosterone both have an influence on neurogenesis. Higher estrogen levels bring increased neurogenesis as do higher testosterone levels. [28, 29]

Attention, Men: Read This Section Closely!

Strikingly, male rats' neurogenesis increased with sexual activity, but female rates of neurogenesis increased only when the female rats controlled the timing of the sexual encounter. When the females did not control the timing, no increase in neurogenesis occurred for them when mating. [14]

The implications of this are profound. Of course humans are more influenced by emotional factors than mice, so some of these data may apply as much to men (at least to some men) as to women. **Emotional attunement is a critical factor in sex.** Rushing through sex faster than one partner wants may leave neurogenesis levels untouched for that partner (although probably most people don't have sex simply to increase neurogenesis).

It's also simply part of being a good lover: mutuality rocks. Don't rush. Wait for each person to be ready for the next step. Optimally both partners feel like they have control in the situation. This will insure that both people get a boost in neurogenesis from making love.

From Couplehood to Parenthood

Elizabeth Gould, Ph.D., is a neuroscience professor at Princeton who's spent most of her career researching neurogenesis. She is currently investigating the effects of parenting on neurogenesis, particularly the processes by which experience as well as certain hormones increase neurogenesis, and how adverse, stressful stimuli reduce neurogenesis.

When Dr. Gould first discovered that oxytocin increases neurogenesis, she naturally assumed that parenting would be one avenue of love that would enhance neurogenesis. However, she soon learned that this assumption was wrong, due to the complex nature of being a parent.

Even pregnancy, so often filled with feelings of happiness, love, and hope, is stressful. During pregnancy brain size decreases, but it returns to normal after delivery. [16] Neurogenesis also decreases during pregnancy in most mammals. [17]

Being a parent is one of the most fulfilling things in life. However, as every parent will attest, it is also stressful. Despite the fact that parenting involves much complexity and rewarding interactions—things that would normally be thought to increase neurogenesis—the research shows that the stresses of parenthood, for both mothers and fathers, seems to outweigh the benefits in terms of neurogenesis. Being an involved parent decreases neurogenesis. [10-13,18] For an uninvolved father, however, this is not the case. [19]

Loving, Supportive Friendships

While oxytocin is neuroprotective against stress, when the stress levels are too high, even oxytocin cannot protect fully, as in parenting. But this helps us understand why loving, supportive relationships are so important. They boost neurogenesis and help protect against stress by buffering its deleterious effects. Just like the monkey in experiment #3, loving friends, supportive co-workers, teachers, mentors, and peers are crucial in dealing with the stress of everyday life.

It's easy to take our friends for granted. We get used to being around our co-workers or family members or neighbors. **We live in an invisible web of relationships.** Most of us hardly realize how important our interpersonal worlds are to feeling good.

Our unique web of relationships holds us. It nurtures us, allows us to be seen, understood, responded to, and cared for. The depth psychoanalyst Heinz Kohut, M.D., once compared our need for supportive, loving relationships to our need for oxygen. Without oxygen we soon die. Without good relationships, after even just a week of isolation, our self structure becomes fragile and fragmented. We become more anxious, shame-prone, vulnerable to the slightest jolt. Good relationships keep our selves strong, cohesive, resilient.

We *can't* **do it alone.** Up until the 1960s or '70s psychology held out an ideal of psychological independence and autonomy that is now seen as wildly unrealistic and altogether wrong. As psychology has deepened its understanding of the psyche, we now see that **people are fundamentally relational.** It is only through relationships that we grow and individuate. Individuation is not opposed to our need for relationships but dependent upon it. We may not be dependent upon any one relationship, but we're interdependent with other people. We become our fullest selves in and through our relationships.

We need other people. We need other people to help us feel good, to integrate our emotions, to help us regulate stress, to help us feel better when we're down, to love, and be loved by. We can live alone if necessary, but it comes at a huge emotional and physical cost. People are an essential part of an enriched environment, the most essential part.

We need a range of relationships. Our selves are complex and multi-faceted. We have a variety of sub-personalities. Different parts of us require different kinds of emotional nourishment, different kinds of relationships. Some of the most common kinds of relationships we need are:

- a lover
- close, intimate friends we can be vulnerable with
- supportive co-workers
- neighbors, peers, family members
- teachers, mentors, guides, role models

Love is the self's most basic nutrient, and it comes in many forms. **When we have a variety of loving relationships, all parts of us can thrive.**

By now there is a vast amount of research data confirming how important good relationships are for our emotional and physical health. The field of psychoneuroimmunology is replete with studies detailing how our immune system is strengthened by loving, supportive relationships and how their opposite weakens our immunity. The field of positive psychology has come to the same conclusions for our emotional health. Positive relationships produce positive states of health and well-being. [27, 38, 39]

The more love in our lives, the higher our neurogenesis is. Doesn't it make sense that our brains grow with love?

Reducing Negative Relationships and Feeling States

There is a great deal of evidence showing that negative relationships impair neurogenesis. If they are bad enough or if the stress is intense enough they can be neurotoxic and can kill brain cells. [44, 46, 49, 50, 29, 30]

There is "good" stress and "bad" stress. Good stress is moderate and temporary. Bad stress is high intensity or chronic stress. Just like exercising stresses your muscles and makes you stronger, so short-term emotional stress builds you up, brings forth new resources, and makes you stronger. Chronic stress, on the other hand, is dangerous in the same way constant, continuous exercise is—it erodes your strength and finally destroys muscle tissue. In the same way, acute (short-term) stress can give your brain a boost and increase neurogenesis. But chronic stress slows down neurogenesis and can become neurotoxic.

When we apply this to relationships it can get confusing, for relationships are both a source of stress as well as a key support that protects from stress. We want to develop those relationships that protect from stress and reduce those relationships that produce stress.

Types of Stressful Relationships

Relationships that chronically engender fear, anxiety, anger, or shame tend to be stressful. Whether it's a critical teacher, a bully co-worker, a controlling lover, a domineering boss, or an acquaintance who's a relentless 1-Up player, stressful relationships hurt both our hearts and our brains.

A single episode of being humiliated or bullied does not shrink our brains, otherwise everyone would be damaged. Generally it takes repeated, continual exposure to a toxic relationship to slow neurogenesis and create the kind of stress that leads to brain shrinkage, impaired immunity, and depression. The earlier in life this occurs, generally, the greater the damage. Childhood sexual or physical abuse can sometimes produce lifelong changes in brain structure, including a shrunken hippocampus, in addition to chronic PTSD.

At this point we don't know how much or how little is needed to start shutting down neurogenesis. Different people have different sensitivities, just as some people are more resilient to stress than others. Indeed, some people emerge from a stressful experience stronger while others suffer PTSD and permanent anxiety from the same event. **But it's clear that chronically stressful relationships are bad for our brains.**

Severe stress can kill brain cells. [49, 50] Newly formed neurons are most susceptible to stress, and these appear to be the first to die in severe social stress.

Being in a dominant vs. a subordinate position in social settings plays an important role in neurogenesis. When you put a bunch of baboons together, they soon form a dominance hierarchy. **Those at the top of the hierarchy have the least stress and show increased neurogenesis.** Those at the bottom have reduced neurogenesis, reduced immunity, higher heart disease, and more depression. [7, 26, 27]

Even more dramatic is the research on bullying or "social defeat." When a mouse or a monkey is forced to live next to an aggressive bully, stress and depression set in while neurogenesis slows down. [24] Repeated, chronic social defeat has strong negative consequences for neurogenesis as well as immunity and depression. [25]

When there's no escape from a tormentor, the only alternative is to shut down and turn off. Neurogenesis also shuts down and turns almost off. Think of being a senior who is partially incapacitated and stuck in a nursing home with an abusive staff. There is no way out. Of course depression rates increase in such circumstances.

Being on the lower end of the dominance hierarchy slows neurogenesis due to a number of mechanisms. Subordinate males have lower testosterone levels, and reducing testosterone is one way to reduce neurogenesis. Subordinate members also have higher levels of stress hormones such as glucocorticoids. High glucocorticoid levels also turn down neurogenesis. Some subordinate members with higher stress levels become depressed, which is also associated with lower neurogenesis. And of course things like hopelessness, despair, pessimism, helplessness—all these reduce immunity, elevate glucocorticoids, and further depress neurogenesis.

A classic study in Britain by Professor Michael Marmot looked at 18,000 men in the British Civil Service over a 40-year period. Those in the higher grades of service had better health, whereas those in the lower grades had lower levels of health and higher rates of mortality. There was a "social gradient" for health. Studies with women later showed similar results. [48]

Being in the top of the socio-economic hierarchy probably is a neurogenic boost. But for those in the lower portion of the socio-economic hierarchy, the results on neurogenesis are not good.

Social instability is another form of social stress that decreases neurogenesis. When the social rules are in flux or when we are thrust into ever-changing new social environments and have too much new social reality to interpret, neurogenesis slows. [8] Rapidly changing job or social situations don't allow a stable dominance hierarchy to form, so we don't know our "places" in the social order. This constant stress of unstable relationships (think about being an immigrant or refugee in a new country) takes a toll on the brain. A certain degree of stability, safety, and security is helpful for maintaining neurogenesis.

Chronic Anger and Hostility—Bad for Your Brain

Another line of research shows that chronic feelings of anger, hostility, rage, and irritation are bad for your brain, your heart, and probably reduce neurogenesis as well. People and baboons with chronic hostility, anger, or rage-proneness show increased heart and cardiovascular disease as a result of an overstimulated stress system.

The high levels of stress hormones and glucocorticoids that chronic anger produces are precisely the same profile that accompanies lowered neurogenesis. [27, 41] Although we can't yet say with absolute certainty that chronic anger and hostility lower neurogenesis, we can infer this with a high degree of probability. If we have a hair-trigger anger response, or even if we are around someone who does, it's helpful to get some distance from this default anger response.

Psychotherapy is remarkably effective at helping people become less angry and to get angry at the right things rather than have a generalized anger response. If you're in a relationship with someone who is a "rage-aholic," encouraging them to get help will save both your brains from needless wear.

People Aren't Monkeys, But We Are Animals

Translating all this into human terms may seem relatively straightforward. Those people who are marginalized by society, discriminated against, or have lower socioeconomic status will have more stress, more illness, and lowered neurogenesis. Mostly this is true. However, there is more to the story.

People have different dimensions of identity, called intersectionality, so that while an abusive boss at work may be stressful for a woman, she may also be a yoga teacher at night who is highly regarded by her students. Being poor may be a choice for a starving artist who gets more meaning from creating his art than making money. Being a valued grandparent who helps look after a couple generations of kids may offset being old and ignored in the rest of daily life. A strong inner meditative and religious life may make being financially poor seem like a minor inconvenience. Or being poor now can be temporarily tolerable when a person believes that much better fortune is coming in the future.

Human beings can cope with stress in ways that baboons cannot. Our beliefs, our capacity to find counterbalancing experiences and alternate sources of nourishment, our ability to create predictability and achieve a sense of control make it hard to make any absolute pronouncements. **People vary in the amount of inner resources they have available to them.** What is true for most people isn't true for everyone.

Lowering chronic stress is critical for brain health and increasing neurogenesis. There are many places to learn more about stress reduction, and below is but a summary of what is necessary.

First, it's important to take some kind of break to focus on something else so the body can return to homeostatic balance. Exercise, a yoga class, a camping trip, an afternoon in nature, a meditation class, square dancing, music—anything you enjoy and can lose yourself in helps the body relax and let go of tension.

Second, incorporate as much as possible of the following:

- Control. Loss of control in a situation is stressful. Focus on ways to achieve some degree of control in your stressful situation.
- Predictability. See if you can increase predictive information such as when and how long this will go on, how intense it will be, what might happen, etc.
- Interpretation of your situation and framing it as important or peripheral.

- Optimism. If you can foresee things getting better, this helps. When you see things only getting worse, this increases stress.
- Social support. Just like the monkey in experiment #1, we need social support to help buffer stress. It needs to be genuine support, from those who really care about us.
- Relaxation response. The body needs to return to homeostatic balance, rest, and relaxation. Learn to relax tense muscles, reduce stimulants, practice meditation, yoga, or other relaxing disciplines.
- Exercise. Aerobic exercise stimulates the body and then allows the body to return to a healthy homeostatic balance. Other forms of exercise such as strength training or stretching are also helpful.
- Unplug from electronics. Being always online produces digital stress that alters your nervous system. Take a break and allow your nervous system to re-set and find its own rhythm, apart from the fast frequency of cell phones, tablets, and computers.

While there is hope for better coping strategies in any situation, the reality of chronic stress, fear, intimidation, anger, and hurt that result from negative relationships impairs neurogenesis. Even though a person can compensate for stressful relationships and mitigate to some extent their toxic effects, such compensations only reduce the negative impact. The positive potential for increasing neurogenesis is lost. Far better is to reduce these kinds of relationships in our lives.

Toxic relationships poison our brains. One recent study showed that stressful relationships—whether with spouses, children, co-workers, or neighbors—resulted in much higher death rates. [45] The answer is not to withdraw from all relationships, for the stress of isolation is roughly equal to the stress of negative relationships. Ideally we want to minimize toxic relationships and maximize positive relationships.

Isolation and Loneliness

Humans are hardwired for relationships. Positive, loving relationships in childhood and adulthood are associated with better health, increased immunity, and greater life satisfaction. People in loving romantic relationships or with close friends live longer than people who are single and isolated. [27] Disruption of social bonds and loneliness are greater risk factors for high blood pressure and cardiovascular disease than smoking or diet. [40]

Social creatures such as mammals, and especially primates, have relationships built into their DNA. There is now massive scientific literature showing how important relationships are to the brain and psyche. Research from different fields—including developmental psychology, infant research, interpersonal neurobiology, depth psychology, and psychopathology research—shows that human beings are fundamentally relational creatures. Success in life is tied to social intelligence more than any other factor. [23] The inability to form relationships is diagnostic in many psychological disorders, including autism, schizophrenia, and other psychoses.

While stressful relationships are hard, at least the person is relating to someone. Being alone and lonely is a whole other kind of deprivation. Short-term isolation is the kind of moderate, brief stress that can either not affect or even increase neurogenesis. **Longer-term isolation powerfully decreases neurogenesis.**

Several kinds of mammals show reduced neurogenesis after chronic isolation. [22]

When isolation and lack of social contact occurs in childhood, the effects are even more devastating on neurogenesis, however, neurogenesis can be restored by then providing social contact once again. [47]

The immensely destructive effects of social isolation cannot be overcome by the most potent neurogenesis stimulator known. As I hope the reader doesn't get too tired of hearing, the most powerful booster of neurogenesis is aerobic exercise. But even running and aerobic exercise do not increase neurogenesis in isolated rats. [5, 6]

There is so much positive stimulation we receive from our relationships. They provide stimulation on physical, emotional, mental, and spiritual levels, bringing complexity and new learning to each encounter. Relationships increase our self-esteem, help us modulate stress, allow us to feel part of the human community, and make us feel good, appreciated, loved. Without this essential nutrient, we wither up emotionally. Neurogenesis slows down as our hearts contract.

Future Dreams

Emotional education will be part of every child's life, starting in the first grade. Working through conflict and anger constructively, learning to become emotionally vulnerable and intimate with close friends and family, deepening the capacity for love and empathy will be prized skills that allow everyone to feel emotionally connected. As a result of this increased emotional awareness, child abuse in all forms no will no longer exist, and when trauma or great stress occurs it will be immediately attended to and worked through.

One-upmanship will be a relic of a bygone era, as will wars, which humanity will have outgrown, and even though there will be hierarchies in organizations this will be accompanied by perfect equality in valuing each person at all levels. Accumulating and hoarding great wealth for oneself will be considered a childish indulgence that no longer occurs as people will strive to actualize their potentials while working for the common good.

Summary

The take-away message of this chapter is: **feeling good and good relationships stimulate neurogenesis while feeling bad and bad relationships reduce it.** We need to do what we can to skillfully move toward authentically loving, supportive relationships and satisfying work and play, just as we need to skillfully transform or reduce negative relationships, work, and play.

One review of the neuroscience research in this area put it this way: "It seems that acute and chronic sociosexual interactions, as positive stimuli, facilitate cell proliferation and survival across distinct brain regions; whereas aversive social interactions leading to psychosocial stress impair adult neurogenesis." [18] I couldn't have put it better myself.

CHAPTER 6

MIND

The human mind is the crown jewel of evolution. Science, art, culture, language, and a complex, well-developed self are some of the mind's highest attainments. The mind makes us human.

When we learn new things, the mind is stimulated and neurogenesis increases. [10] By reading this book and learning about neurogenesis you are increasing your rate of neurogenesis right now.

New learning is part of the "enriched environment" that allows recently created neurons to survive and thrive. For humans an enriched environment consists of physical, emotional, mental, and spiritual stimulation. All are needed for the brain's full development. But mental stimulation has a special place in this fourfold practice, for humanity is, in Aristotle's words, "the rational creature."

Actively engaging our minds pays off doubly: first, by promoting neurogenesis and second, by enlarging our world. When we learn new things about our world it expands our outlook and gives us a wider perspective on life.

Nowhere is the adage "use it or lose it" more true than with our minds. Cognitive testing shows there is a drop-off in mental abilities at two key points in life:

- after leaving school
- after retiring from work

Using our minds less is what both these points have in common. When we slow down our mental engagement, we slow down our minds and neurogenesis. But note: **not everyone experiences such a decline.** Those people who continue to be mentally engaged *do not* see a cognitive decline at these times.

Of course we want to sharpen our mental abilities as much as possible and to stay sharp and alert for as long as possible. Research now shows that almost all cognitive decline is preventable. Some people in their nineties stay clear, focused, and sharp as a tack, with no evidence of cognitive decline. Lifestyle factors greatly outweigh genetics in this. And while starting earlier in life is better than later, it's never too late to stimulate your mind, grow new neurons, and strengthen your cognitive capacities.

Jim

Jim was in his late forties and had a successful career in high tech over the past two decades. "Lately," he began, "I've been off my game. I don't feel as sharp as I once was. Some of the twenty- and thirty-year-olds in my company are nipping at my heels. The tech industry is a young person's game, and it's depressing to think I've aged out of this field I love."

His depression had been increasing over the last six months, though he kept it hidden from his co-workers. "It's harder to get out of bed. My memory isn't holding things as well. At times I can't even force myself to work and just sit in front of the screen surfing the web. This can't go on. I'm getting desperate."

We looked at all aspects of his life. He agreed to start an exercise program, to change his diet along the lines of this book, and to take some time each day for meditation as a stress-reduction strategy. What stood out, however, was how disengaged he felt from his work. He'd always told himself that it didn't matter what project he was on; it was the technical problems he enjoyed. But as he shared more, it became clear that he'd allowed his career to drift into an area he had zero interest in. The mental stimulation of his job was meaningless and boring.

We talked about what he'd need to do to make a mid-career course correction. He was passionate about an area he'd left years before—mapping, technically known as geographical information systems, or GIS. When he thought about returning to it, his face lit up. "I can get my company to pay for some trainings to get me back up to speed," he said. "It'll take some time, but I'm excited to think about moving in this direction again."

Six months later, he was a changed man. "I can hardly wait to get to work in the morning," he said one day. "I never realized how important it was to be excited by my work. I'm sure exercising more and eating better are helping, but using my mind in GIS just feels soooo good," he said with a smile. "Challenging my mind this way is exciting. In some ways I feel more on top of my game than I ever have. It's like I've gotten my mind back."

Mental Functions

To discover the best practices for the mind to increase neurogenesis, let's first review the main mental functions we use daily and need to keep sharp. These include:

- executive function (such as problem solving, planning, inhibition, reasoning, working memory, flexibility, decision making)
- memory (short-term and long-term)
- emotion regulation
- attention and focus
- fluid intelligence
- crystallized intelligence

These terms need some explanation, so let's take a closer look.

Executive function. This comes from the most recently evolved part of the human brain, the prefrontal cortex, which is part of the neocortex. Executive function allows us to plan for the future, to postpone immediate gratification for the sake of greater gratification at a later time (for example, building a business or going to college). Executive function lets us juggle different factors to find the best solution. It inhibits our tendencies to act on impulse and allows us to reason, figure out the best course of action, and then to take that optimal course.

Working memory. This lets us act mentally on several things we are simultaneously holding in memory. For example, I know I have several errands to do: shop for groceries; stop at the drugstore, bank, and cleaners; pick up something from a friend's house; and get gas. I imagine the most efficient route to take to accomplish my tasks, keeping in mind I need to get groceries last so the wild salmon doesn't sit in the hot car all afternoon. Working memory allows me to hold these things in mind as I run these errands.

Working memory lets us keep several pieces of information in mind and manipulate them as needed. It's a short-term process with limited capacity that is easily overwhelmed by anxiety or stress. In working memory we are able to work on the details of the information. While it is a separate cognitive function, it has been linked to other measures of cognitive ability such as intelligence and attention. [10]

Memory, short and long term. Our short-term memory is like a scratch pad, we hold information here for a short period of time, generally about 20–30 seconds. Most people can hold about seven items in short-term memory, plus or minus two. Long-term memory, by contrast, can hold a vast amount of information, but first it needs to be transferred from short-term to long-term memory. Long-term memory consists of explicit (declarative) memory, which is what we can consciously recall at any time, and implicit (procedural) memory, which helps us perform many activities without being consciously aware of it.

Emotion regulation. Emotion regulation is acting in ways to make us feel better and decrease feeling bad. It includes the capacities for self-soothing and self-calming, which regulate how we experience stress, anxiety, shame, and anger. It allows us to tolerate a feeling without either acting it out or repressing it, and to use our emotions as important sources of information and guidance when determining which feelings to act on and which feelings to hold back.

Attention and focus. Attention can be diffuse and global, like a floodlight, or tight and focused, like a spotlight. The ability to concentrate attention and keep it focused is necessary for accomplishing just about anything in life. More complex tasks require a greater capacity for sustained focus and attention, whereas conditions like ADD and ADHD (attention deficit disorder and attention deficit hyperactivity disorder) indicate impairments in the ability to concentrate and focus attention.

Fluid intelligence. Fluid intelligence operates independently of acquired knowledge so we can cope with and creatively adapt to new situations. It allows us to grasp the essence of different conditions so we can see patterns, logically think through issues, and solve novel problems.

Crystallized intelligence. This is the ability to make use of our experiences and acquired knowledge. It includes our accumulated vocabularies and overall knowledge. It improves with age since our store of knowledge increases through experience.

Most IQ tests, such as the widely used WAIS (Wechsler Adult Intelligence Scale) measure both fluid and crystallized intelligence. Although these are two separate forms of intelligence, they are correlated with each other.

These Functions Act Together

These brain functions allow people to go about their complex lives, manage a great many relationships, tasks, desires, perceptions, memories, fantasies, and thoughts throughout the day. We take for granted these astonishing mental feats. They endow the ordinary person with a mind capable of extraordinary comprehension, able to navigate inner and outer worlds of great complexity.

There is a dynamic interplay between the mind's various functions. Executive function, for example, requires coordinating a number of different capacities to be effective. It needs working memory to operate so that a number of factors can be held in mind at one time and manipulated to consider various outcomes. It needs fluid intelligence to deal with novel situations and uses crystallized intelligence to make use of accumulated knowledge for problem solving. It needs emotion regulation to stay on task, inhibiting competing desires and impulses while focusing attention on the problem at hand. Both short-term and long-term memory are used throughout these mental processes.

Memory is an organizing matrix throughout all of this. Sometimes it operates silently in the background, holding different possibilities in place. Other times it comes to the foreground and, as the situation changes, actively brings in new factors that had been held back. Memory is a kind of glue that binds many of the mind's functions together.

We see this most clearly when memory fails. In mild cognitive impairment (MCI), memory begins to fail but the person can still function fairly well in daily life. When memory loss increases, however, everything else begins to unravel as well and the person moves toward dementia. There is loss of executive function, emotion regulation, working memory, attention, and focus. When memory goes downhill further, as in Alzheimer's, the person may even lose touch with who they are, and be unable to recognize family, friends, or even themselves.

Memory is key. **Memory provides an ongoing sense of ourselves that is continuous in time and space.** The whole self crumbles as memory vanishes and our sense of continuity disappears. Dementia is the result. The word "dementia" comes from Latin "de" (without) and "mens" (mind)—"without mind," or overall loss of cognitive ability and the mind's functions.

The Hippocampus Organizes New Memory

The hippocampus is responsible for organizing new memories in the brain. It also acts as a kind of processing center for the formation of new memory; it allows short-term memory to be transferred into long-term memory. Without the hippocampus, explicit new memories are not formed.

The hippocampus is the main brain system for organizing and consolidating new memory, and neurogenesis is essential to keep it functioning at a high level. In both Alzheimer's and mild cognitive impairment, the hippocampus shrinks. To avoid this and keep our memories and minds strong, neurogenesis needs to stay at a high rate. Neurogenesis and memory go together. Increasing neurogenesis increases memory and cognitive function. Mice that have boosted neurogenesis show strong cognitive and memory gains over mice without this neurogenic boost.

Increases and Decreases in Cognitive Functions as We Age

The mental functions listed above vary with age. Once the brain is fully developed, by our early or mid-twenties, some functions get better while others decline as we grow older.

Crystallized intelligence, emotion regulation, vocabulary and language skills, the ability to see things from multiple perspectives, higher reasoning and seeing the limits of knowledge are abilities that generally improve with each passing decade. There is much individual variation in this, however, as some people neglect their minds, causing these abilities to fail to develop or even to diminish. But in general these cognitive capacities increase with age.

On the other hand, fluid intelligence, processing speed, focused attention, and working memory gradually slow down with aging, so our capacity to process new, complex information diminishes slightly with age. Here again there is great individual variation, and those who have practiced some of these skills may show improvements in such things as focused attention, inhibition, and flexibility.

Research done on "average" or "normal" aging shows a gradual diminishing of these functions, corresponding to a decrease in neurogenesis. However, research confirms that mental functions can stay strong into old age, just as neurogenesis can be impressively increased well into very old age.

Here we again encounter the limitations of animal research. Testing on non-human mammals only goes so far, for only human beings read, do long division, and plan for retirement.

To test whether reading increases neurogenesis scientists need to rely on brain imaging, blood flow, performance testing, and post-mortem studies. While this generally makes clear whether or not neurogenesis is occurring, it is indirect evidence. Still, all this evidence points in the direction of increased neurogenesis from discrete areas of learning.

What Are Cognitive Decline and Mild Cognitive Impairment?

We take our mental abilities for granted. But when someone we know develops Alzheimer's, we can see just how central our mental faculties and memory are to the fabric of the self. Indeed, when our minds deteriorate, the very sense of self begins to crumble. This usually proceeds in stages. [1,2]

Cognitive decline means deterioration in cognitive function. Mild cognitive impairment (MCI) is an intermediate stage between the usual cognitive decline of "normal" aging and the more serious decline of dementia. It typically involves problems with memory, language, judgment, and thinking.

MCI is now seen as a transition state toward Alzheimer's and other forms of dementia. Not everyone progresses to Alzheimer's, however. About half progress to Alzheimer's disease within three to five years, a conversion rate of 10–15% per year, depending upon the study. [3,4] Some people die before declining further, and some are diagnosed with other conditions that, when cleared up, resolve the MCI. Of those who survive for ten years, over 90% are diagnosed with Alzheimer's or other dementias.

The most common form of MCI is memory loss, called "amnestic MCI," and it is this form that is generally degenerative and leads to Alzheimer's.

These are the stages of cognitive decline:

Stage 1 is **normal function** (no impairment or memory loss).

Stage 2 is **very mild cognitive decline**, also called **normal aged forgetfulness,** and consists of forgetting names and where things are placed but no loss of functioning. It has recently been discovered that the first part of memory to go for most people is names. The memory for proper nouns is most vulnerable to forgetting because the links are completely arbitrary. Linking a particular name to a particular face is an arbitrary association. This stage consists of "senior moments" but no impairment in daily life.

Stage 3 is **mild decline** or **early confusion.** As memory loss progresses it begins to interfere with work and social situations. Forgetting meetings, customers, or client requests reveals to others that job performance is deteriorating. The person begins to feel anxious and tries harder to carry out tasks that seem too complex and difficult. About 40% of people never progress beyond this point and are fine after withdrawing from situations that are too complex. They die before further deterioration occurs. But 60% continue to decline as MCI transitions into Alzheimer's or another form of dementia.

Stage 4 is **moderate decline** or **late confusion.** Here symptoms of early Alzheimer's disease start to show. Routine jobs like shopping or banking become too overwhelming. There is an impaired ability to do challenging arithmetic, such as counting backward from 100 by 7s. The person forgets personal history and recent events and may become moody or withdrawn.

Stage 5 is **moderately severe decline** or **mid-stage Alzheimer's disease.** Here the person needs help with everyday activities. People at this stage may forget the high school they attended or their addresses. Counting backward from 20 by 2s presents difficulty. People can eat and use the bathroom on their own but may need help dressing properly for the season or situation.

Stage 6 is **severe cognitive decline** or **mid-stage Alzheimer's.** Here people lose awareness of their surroundings, tend to wander and get lost, forget much of their own personal histories, and may have a hard time remembering the names of their spouses or caregivers. Loss of bladder or bowel control is common, and getting dressed often requires help.

Stage 7 is **very severe cognitive decline** or **late-stage Alzheimer's.** At this last stage of mental deterioration people can no longer respond to their environments or have a conversation. Personal care, from eating to going to the toilet, requires help. The person may no longer be able to sit without help or even to smile. Interestingly, music is one of the final forms of memory to go. Some people at this stage still enjoy music and songs from their youth but very little else.

An Ounce of Prevention Is Worth a Pound of Cure

Alzheimer's, dementia, and other end stages of cognitive decline do not present a pretty picture. Current thinking is that by the time symptoms show up, there is already so much damage to the brain that repair is not possible. Even preventing further decline has proven elusive, as the downhill momentum is so strong that no medication yet discovered can hold back the descent into deeper dementia by more than a few months.

This is why adopting a neurohealthy lifestyle as early in life as possible is crucial. Prevention is the better strategy, in fact may be the only strategy. Early detection is seen by many as too late. The time to begin is before the downhill cascade starts. This means increasing neurogenesis and cognitive reserve as early in life as possible.

Just because nothing has yet been discovered that can cure Alzheimer's or restore lost brain function or even slow the decline appreciably does not mean that it's impossible. Integrated, holistic combinations of diet, exercise, and environmental enrichment methodologies that engage body, heart, mind, and spirit have hardly been investigated in clinical trials, mainly because there is no money to be made utilizing natural approaches that don't involve patents on proprietary drugs.

One small pilot study that takes steps in this direction and reported earlier in Chapter Two, researched under the sponsorship of the non-profit Buck Foundation in California, did show improvements in memory in Alzheimer's patients using a non-pharmaceutical approach. It involved dietary and exercise recommendations suggested in this book, such as exercising four to six days a week, taking omega-3s, melatonin and vitamin D, eliminating sugar, getting better sleep, and intermittent fasting.

This was reported in the October 2014 issue of the online journal *Aging*. It is the first holistic approach to research in this area, and its results made headlines in national papers. Hopefully this is just the beginning of such holistic approaches to brain health.

Cognitive Reserve as Brain Protection

One proven way to extend cognitive function is by building what's called "cognitive reserve." This refers to building up the brain by mental exercises—reading, writing, higher education, teaching, professional, and other kinds of complex work. As a result more synapses and connections are formed between different areas of the brain as neurogenesis is stimulated throughout the lifespan.

The concept of "cognitive reserve" grew after some startling results were announced from an early study of a group of elderly nuns' brains after they died. **Researchers discovered that the nuns who had been teachers had the lowest rates of Alzheimer's.** The surprising finding in studying the brains of this group was that many of the teachers had just as much amyloid plaque and neurofibrillary tangles as those with advanced Alzheimer's.

The brains of the teachers looked indistinguishable from the brains of those that had Alzheimer's. But, it was theorized, because this group had used their minds by reading, writing, and teaching their whole lives, their brains had developed more connectivity between various regions of the brain. **They had built up "cognitive reserve" that was used as backup systems to keep the brain functioning well beyond what other brains did.** Much like using alternate fiber pathways on the Internet to get a message through, the brains of these nuns had multiple pathways and connections to get messages through when one pathway got clogged with amyloid plaque.

Since then further research has confirmed these findings and the concept of cognitive reserve has expanded to mean the ability of the mind to resist damage to the brain. In people with equal amounts of amyloid plaque due to Alzheimer's disease, those with lower cognitive reserve show symptoms of Alzheimer's years or decades earlier than those with higher reserve. **Those with higher cognitive reserve have higher brain weights, more neurons, and more complex connections between different areas of the brain.**

When those with higher cognitive reserve do develop symptoms of dementia or Alzheimer's, they decline much more quickly, as the compensatory and backup systems have already been overwhelmed at this point. It is generally a quicker journey to death, but with much less time spent in various stages of dementia since the decline is so rapid.

What Builds Cognitive Reserve?

Not surprisingly, the same things that build cognitive reserve also increase neurogenesis. Those with lower cognitive reserve have a smaller hippocampus; those with higher cognitive reserve have a larger hippocampus. Hippocampal size is directly related to the level of neurogenesis.

The main factors that have been shown to increase cognitive reserve are:

- education (especially higher education)
- type of work (teachers, professionals, high-level executives, and others who use their minds in complex tasks)
- brain size (linked to using cognitive abilities)
- exercise and physical activity
- diet

A study published in 2012 showed that building cognitive reserve from early in life also prevented the buildup of amyloid plaque, the key protein involved in Alzheimer's. This study looked at the specific activities of writing (letters, memos, or emails, for example) and reading (books, magazines, and newspapers). How often someone engaged in reading and writing, especially in the early and middle years of life, directly impacted how much beta-amyloid accumulated in the brain. **The less mental activity, the more amyloid plaque, and the more reading and writing, the less amyloid plaque accumulated.** [5]

Perhaps the most protective effect from cognitive reserve comes from education. A meta-analysis by the National Institute of Health in 2010 concluded that education has a protective effect on the brain by reducing the incidence of Alzheimer's: **the higher the education level, the less the age-related cognitive decline.**

This may be all fine and good for those with formal educations, but what about those who don't have this? What about all those who have been wounded by the problems and limitations of our current educational system and dropped out or stopped participating?

It must be emphasized that education does not necessarily mean formal education like college or graduate school. Yes, going back to school and completing a degree or getting a second degree can be a good idea, even or perhaps especially after retirement. **This points to the importance of lifelong learning.**

But lifelong learning does not require a college or formal schooling. The discipline of college or graduate school is helpful for many people, but the discipline of using your mind to read, study, think, and articulate what's being learned is not confined to a classroom. **Anyone, anywhere can now access tremendous educational resources via the Internet.**

Books, articles, tutorials, webinars, conferences, blogs, discussion groups, video lectures, YouTube, iTunes U, MOOC's, podcasts, and other emerging technologies make anyone's computer or smartphone a more powerful educational source than any university library. All it takes is the intention and discipline to make use of these educational resources.

Given that there is a world of possibilities out there, this leads us to look at what are the types of mental challenges we need to increase neurogenesis.

Mental Practices for Increasing Neurogenesis

It's clear that exercising your mind is the best way to keep it sharp. Learning new things, using your mind to read, listen, explore, inquire—this is the essence of mental stimulation. But while there is agreement about the broad outlines of mental engagement, there is a surprising lack of consensus on what specific activities will help.

I confess that when I started researching this chapter I expected to find many well-designed, replicated studies showing cognitive improvements from certain activities that generalized across the mind. But I found no such thing. Instead I found a research scene closer to the Wild West, where many competing businesses, some founded by entrepreneurial neuroscientists and venture capitalists, jumped on the "brain health" bandwagon to develop specialty computer games and hawk their wares under the guise of science. Much of this literature makes claims that go far beyond the data to make it appear that their particular brand will increase your I.Q. and restore lost brain functions, when in fact there is no evidence to support this.

Most games or activities improve the brain's ability to do that particular game or activity but have no generalizing effect to the rest of the mind. Crossword puzzles, for example, present a very narrow range of mental challenge. This challenge doesn't generalize to other cognitive functions, nor does it even seem to provide much stimulation after the initial few dozen puzzles.

It's similar with working memory. An experiment was run where a college student practiced holding numbers in his mind that were read aloud to him. He practiced this for an hour three to five times a week for a year and a half. At the end of that time he was able to memorize seventy-nine digits in order. But when working memory was tested by substituting letter for numbers, he could only hold six letters at a time in mind. [8]

Most of the research on increasing working memory shows similar negative results. While some studies done with different games or tasks designed to increase working memory show slight improvements immediately after the training, three months later they show no improvement at all. A meta-study of research done in this area confirmed these results, despite what private companies advertise. [7] While green tea has shown to have an increase in working memory, most researchers now believe that working memory is a fixed characteristic, reflecting overall cognitive function that can't be improved through mental effort alone. [7]

Most cognitive activities involve specialized abilities. Doing math problems will stimulate those parts of your brain that process mathematics, but the benefit will not accrue to other parts of the brain. This is the problem with the field of brain enhancement at this time. **Specialized activity, while good in itself, does not generalize to other parts of the brain or help the brain as a whole.** The benefit of challenging mental activities stays in the realm of that particular activity. [6]

This is why almost all programs to increase cognitive reserve, brain health, and neurogenesis are quite limited. Some new research points to very small gains made from video games for older adults that have slight carry-over effects to attention skills when driving, but again the gains are slight.

The solution is to engage in a variety of mentally stimulating activities that challenge a broad range of mental functions. We need both right and left brain stimulation. We need vocabulary, reasoning, and working-memory problem-solving tasks as well as visual-spatial, musical, and intuitive challenges. We need executive function tasks, and we need attention building and concentration challenges. In short, we need to exercise our minds with a wide range of mental activities.

Does Creativity Boost Neurogenesis?

When neurogenesis was first considered as a possibility for some animal species, birds were among the first in which neurogenesis was confirmed. What's noteworthy about this discovery is that neurogenesis in birds is related to their ability to come up with new birdsongs. Birds compose new songs, new themes and variations on themes that depend upon new neurons (neurogenesis). It is one place, therefore, where creativity has been linked to neurogenesis.

The next question is: is this true for humans as well? Does creativity stimulate neurogenesis? At present we don't know. It's interesting to note that exercise increases both neurogenesis and creativity. Exploring how creativity and neurogenesis may be linked is an area for future study.

Another area where human beings differ from animals is bringing meaning into our activities. How does a sense of meaning affect neurogenesis? When our work or actions are felt as deeply meaningful, this acts as an important buffer against stress, so indirectly neurogenesis could be promoted.

Meaning also can make something burdensome feel worthwhile, even joyful. Alternately, when we feel like an activity is meaningless, this brings a sense of alienation that can increase stress. Like creativity, we do not at present know whether meaning increases neurogenesis or whether a lack of meaning suppresses it, but I'd bet on it.

The Brain Drain

One activity that is clearly destructive to the brain is watching too much TV. Passively watching TV for several hours each day is associated with a 20% increased risk for cognitive impairment. [6] The average American watches four hours of TV per day. This is not good for brain health.

Perhaps for someone who is bedridden or confined inside, watching TV provides more mental stimulation than watching the walls for hours on end. But even here, it is better for the brain to also engage in active pursuits such as reading, listening to music, talking, and interacting with others. When brain-impaired individuals are being warehoused in hospitals or old age homes, TV watching may be a humane and even somewhat stimulating form of entertainment. For healthy individuals concerned with brain health, TV watching is best kept within narrow limits as a lifestyle.

Put Your Mind to It

Every brain is one of a kind. What mental practices we need are unique to each of us. Here again there is no "one size fits all" prescription for neurogenesis and brain health. Each of us needs to find our own way. **Each brain requires special nourishment, and we must experiment with different activities to find out what works for us, what we enjoy doing, and what our optimal engagement is.**

When a mental challenge is too difficult, it gets frustrating so we stop. If the challenge is too easy, it gets so boring we stop. Here is another place we need the Goldilocks zone of optimal engagement with mental stimulation so we are interested and excited enough to continue.

It is clear that new learning increases neurogenesis. [10] To maximize this we need to spread it out over different kinds of mental stimulation. What's key is to enjoy this process. We can't do everything, learn every field, or master every discipline. Rather we need to lead with what appeals to us. Lifelong learning is intrinsically rewarding when we follow our interests and pursue what fascinates us.

Practices for the Mind

There are broad categories of mental practices to consider in finding the activities that will enhance our minds.

- **Reading.** This includes different kinds of reading material: fiction (novels and short stories; one neuroscientist says he's hooked on mystery novels), nonfiction (including biography, memoir, self-help, inspirational, travel, books on specific subjects like science or history or neurogenesis), poetry, newspaper articles and magazines, blogs, Facebook and social media posts, Twitter feeds, etc.

- **Writing.** Different kinds of writing include journaling (to put down your thoughts and feelings of the day or week), letters and emails, texts, stories, memos, poems, articles, ads and marketing materials, blog posts, and Facebook updates. The longer the better.
- **Problem solving.** This can be puzzles, board or card games, house repair questions, work problems, life difficulties.
- **Attention and concentration exercises.** Learning to stay focused and on task for hours at a time, concentrating on one problem rather than continually multi-tasking and being distracted by other things, builds our attentional ability. Immersion in a single activity of almost any kind will help this. Meditation, considered in the next chapter, exercises our attention muscles.
- **Executive function tasks.** These involve organizing, planning, executing, following through, and completing complex tasks. They can be part of your work (a special project or ongoing challenge that's part of your job), or just daily projects like shopping, cleaning the house, organizing a party, etc. After retirement when there are less mental challenges, it takes more intention to actively practice working on complex tasks that require executive function. For example, take up cooking if you don't know much about it. Learn about some area you've never entered into before.
- **Discussion groups.** Articulating and expressing our thoughts while also hearing and taking in others' views, adjusting and changing our opinions, simply being in the give-and-take of constructive dialog develops mental flexibility.
- **Musical training.** Learning to play a musical instrument builds up the right brain and those brain regions associated

with playing the instrument. It may also help visuospatial memory and adapting to new information. [6]

- **Video games.** The research is very mixed here. Some research stresses increased violence and aggression after playing violent video games. Other studies have shown that playing certain games results in a slight generalization in ability to process a variety of visual cues.
- **Education.** New learning increases neurogenesis, as a wide variety of studies have shown. Learning can take place in formal or informal settings, the brain doesn't care.

Taking responsibility for our cognitive functioning means exercising our minds. Each of us needs to find the best way to do this.

The results are clear: using our minds to learn, read, write, reason, problem solve, play music, build attention, and increase working memory stimulates neurogenesis, builds cognitive reserve, and protects against Alzheimer's and cognitive decline. Not using our minds decreases neurogenesis and accelerates cognitive decline, memory loss, and Alzheimer's. The choice is ours.

Future Dreams

Once cancer, heart disease, diabetes, and some other common ailments are cured, the average life expectancy will rise to 110, with many people hitting their 120s, some their 130s. People will routinely live full, productive lives into their early 100s, and they will be looked up to as models of wisdom for guidance rather than shunted off into homes for the aged as occurred during the dark ages of the early 21st century.

As society embraces the idea that the highest good is to develop each brain to its highest potential with high rates of neurogenesis for everyone, universal, free public education will allow each mind to progress as far as it naturally wants to, along its unique path. Learning will be a lifelong endeavor, and people of all ages will attend schools of all sorts, not only higher education but schools for particular skills, such as cooking, car repair, gardening, creativity and art schools, physical education programs, emotional education schools, computer programming, teaching schools. Some schools will specialize in students in their sixties, seventies, eighties, and nineties. Many people will get two or three degrees over their lifetimes, reflecting their evolving interests.

Previously scientists in physics and other hard sciences made most major discoveries before they reached thirty-five or so. Since neurogenesis will no longer slow down in the mid-thirties but instead stays high throughout the entire lifespan, major scientific breakthroughs will no longer be limited to the early decades of person's life. Scientific breakthroughs now happen while scientists are in their nineties and one hundreds, which will create a renaissance of new discoveries propelling the human race forward.

With neurogenesis at a higher rate than ever before in human evolution, humanity will operate at a higher level spawning a Golden Age for the world. Cultivating the mind in many different ways will bring a new level of creativity to bear on the world's problems, which will rapidly shrink as new solutions spring forth.

Summary

Exercising the mind by engaging in various forms of mental stimulation increases neurogenesis and keeps mental faculties sharp. There is no quick fix for keeping our mental abilities strong, no one exercise or video game that will prevent the mind from deteriorating. Most forms of mental stimulation are discrete and do not generalize to other parts of cognitive function. Hence, we need to use our minds in as many ways as we can: reading, problem solving, remembering, discussing, writing, musical training, and attention training.

Building cognitive reserve by using our minds throughout our lives is an insurance policy against Alzheimer's and dementia. At whatever age we begin, mental exercise increases neurogenesis and expands our world.

CHAPTER 7

SPIRIT

Because of the materialistic bias in so much of science, very little research gets done on spirituality. Only recently have some neuroscientists investigated the effects of spiritual practices on the brain. What they've found isn't surprising to anyone who has a spiritual practice.

Although to a casual observer it may look like nothing is happening during meditation or prayer—just stillness and quiet sitting—on the inside the experience is powerfully dynamic and creative. This inner dynamism appears to strongly stimulate neurogenesis.

The Early Days of Research

Harvard's Herbert Benson, M.D., was the first to really put meditation research on the map. Benson's initial studies in the 1970s and '80s established that meditation reduces stress and produces a state of relaxation. He began his work investigating a type of mantra meditation called TM (Transcendental Meditation, popularized by Maharishi Mahesh Yogi, though almost all religious traditions use some form of mantra meditation. Mantra meditation is the repetition of a word or phrase over and over again in the mind. The Christian Prayer of the Heart is a form of mantra meditation, for example.)

Benson discovered that regular meditation practice produced a response in the body that activated the parasympathetic nervous system. Although he started his work with mantra meditation, he then broadened his study to include other kinds of meditation practices. All any particular meditation practice needed was a focus, such as a mantra, the breath, or compassion. He, along with others, soon found that most all meditation practices brought about stress relief and relaxation. Along with reduced glucocorticoid and other stress hormone levels, there were higher levels of melatonin and immune system function.

He summarized his findings in his 1975 groundbreaking book, *The Relaxation Response,* which set the stage for further research into different meditation practices along with greater specificity on the physiological effects of these practices on the body and brain. [26] This book also heralded the beginning wave of mind-body research, which demonstrated how "mental" or "emotional" or "spiritual" events have major impacts upon the body and brain.

Mary

Newly retired, Mary had been a mover and a shaker in her career in the corporate world, becoming vice president at a major corporation in her forties and retiring at sixty-five with a reasonable income. However, two years into her retirement, she found herself depressed. "I feel like my brain just isn't working like it used to," she said in our first session. "My life is a lot calmer now than when I was working, but some days I wake up so sad I don't want to get out of bed in the morning."

Mary tried to stay active, and with a good social life she couldn't figure out why she was feeling so depressed. In our work together it appeared she had plenty of mental and emotional stimulation, but she never stopped long enough to actually enjoy what she was doing. An avid golfer, she used golf carts in her outings. One immediate change we made was for her to walk the eighteen holes in her thrice-weekly golf games rather than ride. This provided some much needed exercise.

Focusing on her grief at leaving the work world provided an opening to her emotional life. Discovering that her depression was tied into deep sadness around losing what had been most meaningful to her in her life—her career—allowed her to mourn the end of this phase of her life. As she felt into her profound grief around this loss, other ungrieved losses came up. Gradually, as she let in this pain, the walls around her heart began to melt, revealing a new emotional vulnerability, a side of herself she'd never felt safe enough to show or feel in her corporate life. This heart opening transformed into new vitality and hope, and synchronistically her old Christian beliefs and yearnings from her childhood reignited.

In practicing some heart-centered prayer practices, she found a deeper source of peace inside. And in trying out the mindfulness practices I showed her, she found herself coming alive in a whole new way. "I've been moving so fast in my life that I never took time to look at the sky and the trees when I played golf," she said. "Now I see this really is a time for me to smell the roses and appreciate the present moment I'm in." As her depression lifted and her mind woke up again, the beauty of every new day became a powerful motivation to get up each morning.

What Kinds of Spiritual Practices Work?

There are hundreds of types of spiritual practices among the many religions throughout the world. As research has developed, two key practices have been shown to help brain functioning. Since this field is just in its infancy, there will no doubt be others that future research reveals.

The two main practices that help brain function and appear to stimulate neurogenesis are: mindfulness practices and devotion or compassion practices. What are these practices, how do they work, and why might they increase neurogenesis? To answer these questions, let's make a brief digression into the traditions they come out of to understand why they are so potent.

Two Streams of Spirituality in the World

Spirituality has provided a guiding vision for most every culture throughout history. This universe and everything in it is seen as ultimately a spiritual creation, and only by aligning our lives with this Divine Reality do we find peace, love, and fulfillment. To the extent we are out of alignment, we experience pain, suffering, alienation.

In humankind's upward evolution two major streams of spirituality have emerged around the globe, according to the perennial philosophy. In integral philosophy (another form of the perennial philosophy) these are called traditions of the Personal Divine and traditions of the Impersonal Divine.

The perennial philosophy consists of the core areas of agreement among all the world's religions. [1] It's not that all religions say the same thing—they don't. But they do have a great deal in common and some broad areas of agreement.

Most of the West has developed in traditions of the Personal Divine. Mainstream Christianity, Judaism, and Islam see the Divine as a Personal Being, imaged in the West in primarily masculine terms but imaged in India as male, as female, as both, as neither—but still as a supreme Divine Being. In the nondual traditions, each individual soul is considered a portion of this Divine Being.

In these traditions our souls exist in a relationship of love with this greater Spirit, and spiritual practices use the power of love to bring the soul closer to Divine Union. The soul is our spiritual individuality, beyond ego, an intrinsically joyous, peaceful center of love and light.

Our souls aspire for union with the Divine Beloved, and spiritual practice is designed to purify our outer natures so our souls' deeper love and light can shine through. Love is the path, and spiritual practices work to open the heart to this love. Spiritual practices of love, devotion, surrender, and compassion are central. In some traditional texts of Vedanta, the soul is located in the heart, actually behind the heart chakra on an inner plane.

Much of the East, on the other hand, has been influenced by traditions of the Impersonal Divine. Buddhism, Advaita Vedanta, and Taoism see the Divine not as a Being but as pure Being itself, an infinite Impersonal consciousness, expressed in the three terms: existence, consciousness, bliss (*sat, chit, ananda).* Our fundamental identity in these traditions is identical with that: Buddha-nature, also called the atman (Self) that is Brahman (the Divine.)

Spiritual practices in these traditions of the Impersonal Divine focus on different forms of mindfulness: using the mind's capacity for discernment to free itself from false identifications (ego and its attachments) so that finally the pure spirit shines forth, a universal spirit that is one in essence with all.

It's worth noting that each of the world's religious traditions is quite complex and usually includes the full range of spiritual experience. Thus, mystical Christianity, Kabbalah, and Sufism each speak of the Impersonal Divine even while their main tradition emphasizes the Personal Divine. Similarly, most eastern traditions emphasize the Impersonal but most also include the Personal Divine.

Also, every world religion speaks of an Intermediate plane of existence between this material world and the Divine, a world of angels and demons, ghosts and departed spirits, subtle energies, auras and entities. Shamanism navigates this territory, although shamanic cultures locate themselves within the Personal Divine realm. [28]

Honoring All Traditions

While there has been an ongoing competition between these two streams of spirituality about which one is more "ultimately real," an integral perspective honors both equally. The Divine is both Personal and Impersonal, with neither side privileged over the other.

This allows us to embrace the fullness of our spiritual identity—spirit and soul. We are both a universal spirit (atman, Buddha-nature) that is one with all as well as unique, individualized souls evolving toward greater purity and union with the Divine Being.

Mindfulness and Heartfulness

These two streams of spirituality have developed spiritual practices designed to unveil our deeper spiritual identities, either spirit or soul, depending upon the tradition. Traditions of the Impersonal Divine focus on different approaches to mindfulness to discover the spiritual ground of our beings. Traditions of the Personal Divine focus on what can be called "heartfulness" practices of love, devotion, compassion, or surrender to discover our inmost souls.

It's important not to separate these practices too rigidly. In fact, both practices appear in both traditions, even though the emphasis differs in each. Thus, traditions of the Impersonal Divine that focus on mindfulness see compassion and loving kindness meditation as necessary preliminary practices, for we can only be as mindful as the heart is open. Similarly, traditions of the Personal Divine put their main emphasis upon devotional prayer and bhakti meditation but see the calming of the mind (which can be brought about by mindfulness) as preparatory to opening the heart.

Both practices appear to enhance neurogenesis. Let's look at what's been discovered so far.

The End of Animal Studies

Much of the research on neurogenesis draws on work with non-human mammals. On the physical level this is relatively straightforward: most carcinogens cause cancer with mice, monkeys, and humans; humans share the same neurotransmitters and brain organization with other mammals, so brain changes due to diet or drugs appear to work across species. While there are exceptions to this, by and large it holds true.

On the emotional level, as noted earlier in this book, there is also a large degree of overlap. But humans have a much greater emotional complexity, so we need to be more cautious and tentative in translating mammal data to humans, especially given humans' greater capacity for emotion regulation.

The mental level involves greater checking with human research and data. New learning is helpful for mice and monkey brains as well as humans. But only humans can learn arithmetic, languages, and music, with cognitive skills far beyond all other animals.

When we work with spiritual practices, we enter a realm where we can no longer draw upon animal data. Mice and monkeys, so far as we know, do not meditate or pray. All of the data in this chapter come from human studies, which means there is a greater degree of interpretation, as noted earlier, since we can't do experiments with humans, and then kill them and slice their brains to see what changes occurred. Like much of science, this area is not clear-cut, and there can be honest differences of interpretation.

However, we do know by now that there are strong indications of neurogenesis that can be observed. For example, such biomarkers as increased hippocampal size, increased blood flow to the hippocampus, increased glucose metabolism, increased cognitive performance, lower stress hormones, decreased depression, and increased memory all accompany neurogenesis. Usually when these things are occurring, neurogenesis is occurring. And these data are what we look at in this section.

What Is Mindfulness Meditation?

Mindfulness meditation is the process of training the mind to come increasingly into the here and now. One working definition of mindfulness is "paying attention on purpose." **Different mindfulness practices teach the mind to stop its usual preoccupation with ordinary thinking and daydreaming and to instead wake up and fully attend to the present moment.**

Some practices do this by focusing attention on the sensations of the breath. When attention wanders, the meditator gently brings his or her attention back to the subtle sensations in the body of the breath going in and out. Over time, restless thoughts settle down, and the mind becomes exquisitely focused upon the sensations of breathing. This attentional capacity is then brought into daily life.

Some practices do this by focusing attention on feelings or thoughts. In some forms of meditation, thoughts or feelings are simply labeled "thinking" or "feeling" and then the thought or feeling is let go of. In becoming aware of awareness there is a gradual "waking up" of consciousness into the here and now along with the realization of how much of our daily lives are spent in a kind of semi-conscious trance, almost sleepwalking.

Still other practices focus on the entire contents of consciousness—thoughts, feelings, sensations, images—while holding them all lightly, allowing them to arise and pass away rather than getting drawn into the usual melodrama. In letting everything that comes up pass by, like watching clouds float by in the sky, we discover a deeper center of identity within. **In focusing upon consciousness itself, rather than the contents of consciousness, the internal dust begins to settle and a greater awakening occurs that brings us into a more present-centered state.**

Variations on this theme occur in the Vedantic tradition, where the practice is to draw back into a silent witness consciousness that is separate from the whirl of thoughts, feelings, sensations. From this peaceful inner witness there is a dis-identification with the contents of consciousness and a discovery of a deeper level of our beings.

While the term "mindfulness meditation" and many of its practices come out of the Buddhist tradition, Buddhism's lack of metaphysical beliefs makes this practice applicable to anyone from any tradition. Catholic nuns and monks are incorporating mindfulness meditation, for example, and in fact there are analogous practices in other traditions, though not called by this name.

Throughout all these various practices the person learns how to "be" and to find an inner center of peace and calm amidst the daily activities and incessant "doing" of ordinary life. This is stress reduction *par excellence.*

Mindfulness Meditation and Neurogenesis

Mindfulness meditation is one of the most studied forms of spiritual practice. There are now mindfulness research centers at major universities, including Harvard, Yale, Stanford, UC Berkeley, and UCLA.

One of its first well-researched uses was in stress reduction and pain management. Jon Kabat-Zinn, Ph.D., at the University of Massachusetts, showed that mindfulness meditation training had a powerful effect in reducing stress and pain in chronically ill patients. [2,3] Further research replicated this work and extended it to stress and anxiety in a wide variety of populations. [4]

As research confirmed its use with stress and pain management, it was used with depression, and research showed impressive results. [5,6] Since then it has become increasingly incorporated into psychotherapy, and by now there are hundreds of studies showing its efficacy for such things as ADD, ADHD, increasing empathy, couples therapy, borderline personality disorders, emotion regulation, executive functioning, reduced negative affect, self-esteem, lower pain sensitivity, and enhanced psychological well-being. [4]

The alert reader may have noticed that some of these conditions are related to diminished neurogenesis. **Depression, stress, anxiety, negative affect, and lowered executive function are all implicated in lowered neurogenesis.** So if mindfulness meditation improves these conditions, could it also increase neurogenesis?

Other studies point to this being the case. One thing that goes along with increasing neurogenesis is the hippocampus gets larger. As noted earlier, sometimes the hippocampus increases along the side connected to memory and cognitive abilities, while other things (like antidepressant medication) increase the side connected to emotion regulation, specifically stress and depression regulation.

Mindfulness meditation increases the size of the hippocampus along its entire length. This increase in hippocampal size also goes along with a thickening of cortical structures in some other parts of the brain, especially the prefrontal cortex, but it is the growth in the hippocampus that is most dramatic and which has been the major focus of research. [7, 8] Gray matter (neurons) increases in the hippocampus and parahippocampus result in larger hippocampal volumes globally, larger hippocampal radial distances locally, and in addition there is enhanced connectivity in the white matter pathways. [13-19] All this could simply indicate more synaptic connections being formed, but the dramatic increase in hippocampal size shows that probably more is occurring than just increased synapses. It strongly points to neurogenesis.

The increase in hippocampal size was especially pronounced in long-term meditators. But growth in the hippocampus was even measurable in people who practiced 30 minutes per day in an eight-week training program.

It was surprising to the researchers that even eight weeks of mindfulness resulted in measurable brain changes. This shows how quickly the brain can adapt and change. [9]

Even more striking were the increases in long-term meditators. The amount of increase in gray matter in the hippocampus directly correlates to years of practice of mindfulness meditation practice. There is also more gray matter in other areas of the brain connected to sense of self and empathy. Conversely, there is a decrease in the gray matter of the amygdala, the part of the brain that is always on the alert for fearful or traumatic stimuli. These changes are associated with a decrease in anxiety, fear, and stress.

For neurogenesis to occur, the growing neurons need additional blood supply to nourish the growing cells. So another indirect way to determine if neurogenesis is occurring is to look at the blood supply to the brain, specifically to the hippocampus. **Indeed, after practicing mindfulness, neuroimaging studies confirm that there is an increase of blood flow to the hippocampus—exactly what we'd expect if neurogenesis were occurring.**

Still another line of evidence for neurogenesis comes from studies of mindfulness and increases in working memory and autobiographical memory. As discussed earlier in the section "Practices for the Mind," working memory in particular is extremely difficult to enhance. Almost all claims of memory enhancing programs only work on specific memory centers, not on working memory more globally. Yet mindfulness has been shown to enhance working memory. Increased specificity of autobiographical memory has also been reported. [20-23]

All of these biomarkers are, to be sure, correlated with neurogenesis but not proof. For that we'll need to wait until a number of long-term meditators die and donate their brains to science. But at this point, there are very strong indications that mindfulness practice does stimulate neurogenesis. [13]

In addition, mindfulness brings about synaptic growth in the prefrontal cortex, especially the left portion responsible for executive function, abstract reasoning, emotion regulation, and positive emotions. Mindfulness' ability to bring greater inner harmony, better decision-making, and equanimity are well documented.

Devotion and Compassion Practices

The other main set of spiritual practices from the world's religious traditions is designed to increase love, devotion, compassion, and empathy for all living beings. These devotion and compassion practices can take many different forms.

One practice common to Christian, Islamic, and Vedantic traditions is to have an object of love or devotion, say Jesus or the baby Krishna or the Divine Mother, and to focus on feelings of love, devotion, bhakti, surrender, admiration, appreciation, and adoration toward this being, while simultaneously dis-identifying from negative feelings and impulses. **Over time love and devotion develop from impure forms toward increasing degrees of purity, intensity, and selflessness.** The deeper soul within shines through the external nature and calls on the Divine for union as the soul's peace, light, and love flood the outer self.

Another variation is to concentrate in the heart area on a feeling—love, devotion, surrender, or aspiration for the Divine— while disregarding other feelings and thoughts. Aspiration (different from vital desire) is a calm, peaceful longing of the soul for the Divine, the voice of the evolving soul. The power of aspiration, or love, *bhakti*, devotion opens the gates of the inner heart. As these feelings intensify, the heart opens to a deep interiority and reveals the joy, peace, and love of the luminous soul and the Presence of the Divine.

Another practice that has been well studied from the Buddhist tradition is to begin with oneself, then extend compassion and loving kindness to friends and family, then to others who are suffering or whom the person feels negatively toward, and finally to the entire world.

May I have happiness.

May I be free of suffering.

May I experience joy and ease of being.

Repeat these phrases first toward oneself, then toward close friends and family, then to those in pain, and finally for everyone in the world as the circle of compassion extends outward.

There is much similarity among these practices, all of which are designed to bring forth greater love, compassion, empathy, and caring for others and the earth.

Neurogenesis and Devotion and Compassion Practices

These practices are just starting to be studied and have less research behind them than do traditional mindfulness practices. However, there is great evidence to show that these practices stimulate neurogenesis.

Devotion and compassion practices also bring about a larger hippocampus, increased blood flow, and an increase in positive feelings, empathy, as well as reduced stress, anxiety, and depression. [10, 11, 25] Again, these would be expected if neurogenesis were happening, and the research confirms these effects in humans. However, when we add the hormonal stimulants for neurogenesis to the data below, it amounts to a case even stronger than that for mindfulness that devotion practices increase neurogenesis.

Another line of research comes from the Institute of HeartMath outside Santa Cruz, California. Years of studies on the heart and positive emotions such as love, caring, gratitude, and appreciation show that these emotions have strong stress-reducing effects while increasing immunity and greater coherence of brain waves. [12]

Love, the Ultimate De-Stressor

If love is the highest value of life, as spiritual teachers have said for thousands of years, doesn't it make sense that it's good for us—good for us spiritually, emotionally, and physically by renewing our brains through neurogenesis? **Love and related feelings such as gratitude, devotion, appreciation are hallmarks of spiritual development in all spiritual traditions.**

Researchers at HeartMath institute have found the following:

- Focusing in the heart area for a period of 20–30 seconds brings greater coherence to heart rhythms and brain wave patterns.
- Focusing on a feeling of love, devotion, appreciation, or gratitude while centered in the heart increases the heart-brain coherence.
- It increases the body's immune response as measured by higher IgA levels, a bio-marker of immune system function.
- It decreases stress, as measured by lower glucocorticoid levels and lower blood pressure.
- It increases the so-called youth hormone DHEA. [12]

The chapter on diet shows that DHEA stimulates neurogenesis, and increasing DHEA levels increases neurogenesis.

Further, we know that feelings of love stimulate the release of oxytocin. It is also well-known that oxytocin stimulates neurogenesis. Practices that evoke love and loving feelings (such as devotion, surrender, aspiration, *bhakti*, adoration), which love and devotion practices do, should therefore stimulate neurogenesis.

It has been well established that meditation increases melatonin levels. [24, 27] Melatonin also increases neurogenesis, providing a further avenue by which new neurons are produced.

By increasing oxytocin, melatonin, and DHEA levels, we have three known hormonal stimulants of neurogenesis that are released when doing devotion and compassion practices. Higher levels of these three substances make increased neurogenesis extremely likely. This is considerable evidence for biochemical and hormonal mechanisms for increasing neurogenesis. There may well be other practices not yet known by which states of love, compassion, and devotion produce neurogenic effects.

The Renewal of Spirit

The world's spiritual traditions offer a radical vision of health and renewal. They hold out the realization of mindful awareness and love as continuous states of being, of operating at a higher level of peace and joy in daily living, of love that is inherent in the soul's being, not dependent upon outer circumstances or events.

Mindfulness of everyday life brings us into the eternal Now, with its peace and wide acceptance of what is. This brings relief from the stresses that come with trying to deny reality or imagining more stresses than actually exist. As one Buddhist teacher said, "Pain times resistance equals suffering." Mindfully opening to our present experiences, melts this resistance and the stress it creates.

Feeling love and caring in our interpersonal relationships is an essential part of "the good life," and the chapter on the heart goes into detail explaining why this is the case. But spiritual traditions go even farther.

Spirituality holds out the promise of living continuously in a state of love, beyond any particular human relationship—a love for all creation. This is a state that spiritual practice prepares us for by gradually purifying our nature, from the density of our present experience (desires, attachments, negative feeling states) so we might live in a higher vibration, one attuned to joy, peace, love, and gratefulness.

The renewal of love encompasses the renewal of our brains. Our brains thrive in love, in the peace and joy and freedom from stress that come from deep states of love. When we are in these states, we see that so many of our problems and stresses are the result of our limited consciousness and constricted ways of seeing things.

In the larger vision that comes in deep states of love, most of our daily problems fade away or the solutions become clear. Contracted states of non-love create the very problems we feel stressed by. Love is our deepest identity, and in becoming this we move beyond the anxiety and stress that comprise so much of daily life.

Neuroscience seems to be on the verge of showing us that the great truths of the spiritual traditions are in fact exactly what is most helpful for brain health and renewal.

Future Dreams

As humanity evolves into a Golden Age, people will move beyond their exclusive identification with the body and realize the deeper, inward identity of spirit. In this age people will live in a sense of unity and love for all. There is simultaneously a heightened individuation into each soul's uniqueness and a oneness with others and the cosmos.

Accidents and pain will still be part of life, but with everyone trained in meditation as children, people will soon learn not to resist such things inwardly, which will reduce their stressful impact. All humans will be children of the Divine, brothers and sisters with a shared yet differentiated consciousness.

The nation-state will give way to global governance that eliminates war, food shortages, pollution, and rapacious greed. Social justice will no longer be an issue as humanity grows into a sense of love and caring for all, in which fairness, justice, and the common good will be inherent in every action. Differences will be resolved via higher integrations rather than discord, producing greater harmony and more inclusive understandings.

Within a fathomless inward peace, the vivid, mindful awareness of every moment will make each new day a miracle. Each person's brain will flower in the delight of existence and an enveloping love for all creation. The joy of living will be enhanced by the shared harmony created with others as all people discover new depths and potentials throughout their long, productive lives.

Summary

Two spiritual practices seem to especially promote neurogenesis:

- mindfulness practices, such as meditation
- heart-centered practices, such as love, aspiration, bhakti, devotional prayer, or compassion

Practice over time appears to increase the effects of these disciplines, but as little as eight weeks of daily, half-hour meditation practice produces measurable results. As research continues to investigate the realm of spirituality, it may well discover other spiritual practices that enhance neurogenesis.

CHAPTER 8

INCREASE NEUROGENESIS
BY NOT SLOWING IT DOWN

We know how to dramatically increase neurogenesis to enhance our cognitive abilities and emotional resilience. But to make the most of this opportunity, we need to pay equal attention to what gets in the way. After all, there isn't much point in trying to be healthy if we're poisoning ourselves at the same time. It's a dual strategy we need to follow:

1. Increase neurogenesis and BDNF levels.
2. Stop what decreases neurogenesis and BDNF levels.

Unless we do both our efforts will be like stepping on the gas and brake pedals at the same time. We'll go nowhere fast.

The Four Poisons:
> **Chronic Inflammation**
> **Chronic Stress**
> **Physical Assaults**
> **Deprivation**

Just as science has been studying what increases neurogenesis, researchers have also been learning what slows down neurogenesis and lowers BDNF levels. Most of this book is devoted to foods and activities that are neurohealthy. This chapter focuses on factors that are neurotoxic and best avoided so we don't undo all our gains toward increasing neurogenesis.

Neurotoxins come in many forms. They can be emotional stresses that reduce neurogenesis and kill neurons. They can come from the body's own protective inflammatory response. They even come in the form of a deprived, impoverished environment with minimal sensory stimulation, mental stimulation, and emotional nourishment. All of these slow neurogenesis and drastically reduce the brain's BDNF levels. On top of this, physical assaults, such as mercury poisoning or a sharp blow to the head, can also have debilitating results for the brain.

This list of four poisons isn't exhaustive, but they are the main ones we encounter in daily life. Let's take each poison in turn.

Poison 1: Inflammation

Inflammation is a healthy response to injury or infection. The heat, swelling, and redness from inflammation are part of how the body protects itself. For example, when you cut your finger and get an infection, the body sends white blood cells (macrophages) to find and kill off the invading bacteria. The redness and swelling indicate the body is mounting an attack to repel the invaders. This healing action of the body's immune system keeps us safe from outside marauders and when the foreign bacteria have been killed and cleaned up, the redness subsides.

Inflammation is of two kinds: acute and chronic. Acute inflammation is short-term. It starts with a discrete infection or need to heal a wound, and it ends when the infection is cured or the wound healed. Acute inflammation is essential to health. It focuses the body's defenses against a particular problem.

Chronic inflammation, however, is when the protective cascade doesn't stop or becomes too intense or fails to attack the outside invader and turns on the body instead. This is when inflammation becomes unhealthy. **In chronic inflammation the body turns on itself as inflammatory defenses run amok.**

Chronic inflammation has now become more widely understood to be a serious health threat. It is behind or implicated in seven of the leading causes of death in the US: cancer, stroke, diabetes, nephritis, Alzheimer's, and chronic lower respiratory disease. [1-9] It is a major cause of heart disease. It is central in the autoimmune diseases rheumatoid arthritis and lupus, as well as in Huntington's disease, ALS (Lou Gehrig's disease), and Parkinson's. Even multiple sclerosis (MS) is characterized by chronic inflammation of neural tissue. [10-14]

One big problem with chronic inflammation is that it generally goes unrecognized. It's known as "the silent killer" because it operates out of sight and below awareness. Because it is unnoticed, it can work for years under the surface, slowly killing parts of the body or brain.

Why Inflammation Is Neurotoxic

As part of its inflammatory cascade the body has a number of cells dedicated to finding and attacking invading cells from the outside. Called macrophages, they act like soldiers on "search and destroy" missions, overcoming foreign cells and neutralizing them. In autoimmune diseases such as lupus and rheumatoid arthritis these cells mistakenly attack the body.

In the brain these soldier cells are called microglial cells, and their job is to engulf dead neurons killed by injury or infection. Their armaments consist of neurotoxins and free radicals, which work quite well to neutralize dead neurons and invading bacteria, viruses, and harmful substances. **Unfortunately, when the job is done, the inflammatory defenses often persist, and these very same neurotoxins and free radicals then attack healthy brain cells.**

One indication of chronic brain inflammation is high levels of microglial cells, and neurodegenerative diseases such as Alzheimer's, Parkinson's, Huntington's, MS, and ALS show high microglial activity. [10,11] Other factors that can trigger chronic inflammation include high blood sugar levels, along with emotional and oxidative stress (free radicals). [12]

While research into Alzheimer's disease is progressing, much is unknown. It is clear that beta-amyloid provokes an inflammatory cascade that includes cytokines, microglial activation, and other signaling mechanisms that gradually kill brain cells in large numbers, especially neurons in the hippocampus. Loss of memory, inability to learn, dementia, and eventually death result from these inflammatory processes.

As we age chronic inflammation increases. Cognitive decline in aging is highly correlated with increasing inflammation levels.

Chronic inflammation not only is neurotoxic, it also decreases neurogenesis and inhibits neural plasticity.

One measure of general inflammation throughout the body is a blood test called C-reactive protein. It is helpful to include this test as part of a yearly physical exam. Higher CRP levels indicate high inflammation and are associated with lower brain volume and cognitive decline. [38] Even the chronic inflammation from gum disease (periodontitis) is associated with cognitive decline. [37]

In chronic inflammation the body attacks its own brain cells, shrinking the brain and decreasing neurogenesis. **Reducing inflammation is imperative.** Therefore, we need to see what causes inflammation and what reduces it.

What Causes Chronic Inflammation?

Many things that are part of normal living cause chronic inflammation. These include:

- toxic chemicals such as smog, pesticides, mercury in fish
- smoking, drinking alcohol
- insulin resistance and high blood glucose levels
- free radicals (oxidation)
- obesity and excess fat
- chronic stress of all kinds, including physical and emotional stress
- physical stress, such as not sleeping, colds, gum disease
- emotional stress, such as anxiety, fear, loneliness, depression, isolation, angry relationships, abusive relationships, bullying, rejection, being unemployed or poor, discrimination, being always online and never having downtime to unplug, job insecurity, or abusive bosses or co-workers

In short, many of our everyday life stresses produce the chronic inflammation levels that increase as we age.

This would just be depressing if there were nothing we could do to change it. But there is a great deal we can do to reduce chronic inflammation and protect our brains.

Eliminate or reduce foods, substances, and situations that are pro-inflammatory. Second, eat anti-inflammatory foods, spices, and supplements to reduce your general level of inflammation, as suggested in the chapter on diet. Reduce exposure to chronic stress, excess fat, and toxins such as smoking and alcohol. Check your progress by paying attention to biomarkers of chronic inflammation such as CRP, homocysteine, and fibrinogen blood levels when you get a yearly physical exam to insure inflammation is lowering.

Poison 2: Chronic Stress

We've learned that *acute* inflammation is a healthy response to healing an infection or wound but *chronic* inflammation destroys the very body tissues it was meant to protect. **Stress operates the same way.** *Acute* stress helps energize us to cope with a crisis, but *chronic* stress damages both the body and brain.

Although we think of physical stress and emotional stress as very different things, the body treats both kinds of stress the same way: *it initiates a stress response to try to overcome the stressor.*

Not All Stress Is Created Equal: Good Stress and Bad Stress

Acute stress is evolutionarily adaptive. It supercharges our "fight or flight" circuits. Seeing a lion approach on the African plain, the stress responses of faster heartbeat, hypervigilance, and glucose pouring into the bloodstream to energize muscles to climb safely up a tree kept our ancestors alive. And when the lion moved on, they could come down from the tree and relax. Our bodies are superbly adapted to this kind of short-term stress.

Short-term stress strengthens us. If we don't stress our muscles through exercise, they waste away. If we don't stress our minds by learning new things, our minds atrophy. Facing a difficult emotional challenge brings forth new resources within us, allowing us to grow as people. **Good stress helps us grow stronger.** Then, when the stress is over, our body returns to its homeostatic balance. We relax and chill out.

Good stress increases neurogenesis. It's as if during good stress (short-term, moderate stress) the body sends a signal to the brain that says, "Hey! Wake up! Something's going on that we need to cope with. Make some new brain cells to figure this out—fast!"

Good, short-term, moderate stress (and its accompanying stress hormones) is our friend. It's too simplistic to say we need to lower stress hormones in the body, because we need some stress hormones to make us stronger (and sometimes to increase neurogenesis). [18] Stress hormones help us, except when they don't by being chronic.

Bad Stress

When stress is chronic and doesn't end, it exerts a powerfully destructive effect on the body and brain. **Bad stress is continuing, ongoing stress that never allows the body to return to its natural homeostatic balance.**

We can think of three kinds of stress that relate to our three "brains." All animals experience physical stress, like charging lions or lack of food. Humans' reptilian brain stem responds to this stress by turning on the survival circuits of "fight or flight." When the lions leave or food is found, the stress ends and balance returns to body systems.

In primates there is another kind of stress—social stress. The monkeys at the bottom of the dominance hierarchy experience the most stress. Humans' advanced limbic system (our second "brain") gives us all a good sense of when to flee or when to stand and fight in similar circumstances, whether it's at a high school party or a meeting at work. Here again, when it's over, the body settles down in homeostatic balance.

In humans, however, there is a third type of stress— psychological stress. This comes from our third "brain," the neocortex's ability to anticipate the future and to dwell on the past. Anticipating a public talk is one of the most stressful events people identify. And then, even when it's over, we can dwell on how poorly we did and keep the stress going for a very long time. **Psychological stress becomes chronic stress.**

Additionally, the neocortex is responsible for the sense of self, or ego. We rarely come across a lion charging at us as we come out of Walmart. But we all experience multiple daily assaults on our self-images. When our self-images are threatened, we experience stress, lots of it.

Since almost no one has such a solid, integrated, cohesive sense of self that is bullet-proof against these daily insults, **the interpersonal world becomes an ongoing source of stress.** "Am I good enough? Will I be able to meet this work goal? Will this person like me? Can I get that job? Will my company go under and leave me unemployed? Will the bad or shameful things I've done in my past catch up with me? Will people like me? Can I get over this particular loss? Will I be okay in the future? Will I find someone to love?"

The neocortex, that highpoint of evolution that brings out the greatest human capacities, can also make our lives a chronically stressed hell.

Our brains evolved to deal with the first two kinds of stress pretty well. However, our primate ancestors never had to worry about paying rent or losing their jobs. Chronic psychological stress is new to our bodily systems, and most of us aren't handling it very well yet.

A Brief Overview of How Stress Damages Health

The US National Academy of Sciences reports that *70–80% of all doctor visits are for stress or stress-induced illnesses.* By now there is so much evidence showing that chronic stress damages health that it would take volumes just to show how this works on the molecular level and more volumes to show how it works on the cellular level. **The evidence is overwhelming:** *chronic stress is the major killer of our time.*

The stress hormones released by the body at times of stress are various corticosteroids, including adrenaline, noradrenaline, cortisol, and other glucocorticoids. Over the short term these help the body cope. But long-term exposure to these stress hormones damages major systems of the body:

- The immune system is compromised (since it's more adapted to use the body's energies to flee from the lion than it is to hunt down cancer cells that won't be fatal for several years, hence increased cancer rates) and more susceptible to autoimmune disorders, like asthma and lupus.
- High blood pressure, increased cholesterol, heart, and cardiovascular disease, stroke, heart attack
- Diabetes and insulin resistance [33, 40]

- Reproductive problems and decreased sex drive in men and women as sex hormones are inhibited.
- Osteoporosis in women
- Damage to muscle tissue and tense muscles, leading to headaches, backaches, other muscular pains
- Gum disease
- Growth inhibition
- Stomach and intestinal troubles including ulcers, colitis, IBS
- Weight gain from increased eating
- Mental health issues, especially anxiety, depression, and memory problems

How Chronic Stress Damages the Brain

Chronic stress shrinks the brain, shrivels neurons, decreases neurogenesis and BDNF levels, and has a host of other neurotoxic effects. It appears to even kill some brain cells outright, as it definitely does in animals. [15]

The hippocampus, the site of the brain's neurogenesis that we've been learning so much about in this book, is more endowed with glucocorticoid receptors than any other part of the brain. So it is affected by stress more than any other part of the brain.

From an evolutionary perspective it makes sense to have the hippocampus on high alert at times of stress, so that memories and emotional reactions can be engraved on the brain to guard against similar future threats. If my brain knows that lions roam in this part of the forest and I can escape up these trees, it may save my life again later.

The Incredible Shrinking Brain

The problem comes with *chronic* stress. The accompanying constant glucocorticoid stimulation dramatically decreases the size of the hippocampus and its ability to function. Studies of people with severe chronic stress (such as some forms of PTSD) show that the hippocampus is up to 25% smaller than normal. [15, 16] **Having a hippocampus one quarter smaller means cognitive and memory deficits as well as emotional vulnerabilities.**

Up until recently, researchers knew that stress causes memory problems but didn't know why. Now through MRI and CT brain scans, it's become clear that in extreme stress, and with a hippocampus missing up to one quarter of its mass, it is much harder to form new memories and manage our emotions. Chronic stress withers the branching dendrites of neurons, decreasing their webs of connection to other neurons. New neuron birth is slowed, cell growth is slowed, the entire hippocampus fails to activate like it should to make new memories. [17, 18]

Further, the elevated glucocorticoid levels triggered by chronic stress is toxic to neurons, especially hippocampal neurons. Whereas acute stress floods the brain with glucocorticoids that increase memory, after just half an hour these very same glucocorticoids have the opposite effect and disrupt memory. [39]

To add insult to injury, because the hippocampus is involved in regulating glucocorticoid levels, as it gets damaged it is unable to control the very things that are hurting it. The hippocampus's regulation of glucocorticoids gets thrown out of whack as it loses its ability to turn down or turn off glucocorticoid release. So the whole thing spirals out of control, subjecting the brain to ever higher levels of toxic hormones, which in turn makes it even less able to regulate what's poisoning it, etc., etc. in another downward spiral. So, the worse we get, the worse we get. (This same negative spiral also occurs in Alzheimer's.)

Chronic Stress Increases Inflammation

In just the past few years researchers have come to understand how chronic stress increases inflammation. There are a number of pathways by which stress produces inflammation. Initially, stress hormones can have an anti-inflammatory effect. However, over time the body's immune cells become insensitive to cortisol's regulatory effect on inflammation. Stress causes inflammatory cytokines to be released, and even the brain itself can initiate an inflammatory response to stress. [40]

Stress and Depression

These very same mechanisms are why stress so often leads to depression. If you speed your car you soon run out of gas. *Chronic stress is like keeping your foot on your car's accelerator: you use a lot of gas.* And the body that never gets a chance to rest, replenish, and refuel, soon collapses into depression.

The animal experiments are clear and compelling. Stress any mammal for a little while, and this soon elicits the classic stress response. Keep the stress going so it becomes chronic stress, and the animal soon becomes depressed—resulting in lethargy, loss of appetite, sleep disturbances, weight gain or loss, lack of interest in its surroundings, loss of interest in sex or other pleasures, loss of exploratory behavior. These are all the classic symptoms of depression.

The precise biology of how stress leads to depression is not fully understood, but the basic outline is in place:

- Most depressions are triggered by stressful events.
- High corticosteroid levels in animals and humans create higher risk for depression. Depressed people have higher levels of corticosteroids.
- High levels of stress hormones such as corticosteroids create resistance to their effects which impairs the brain's capacity to regulate these levels.
- Stress lowers neurogenesis, and reduced neurogenesis is central in depression.
- Stress lowers BDNF levels, and lower BDNF levels are a key feature of depression as well as lower neurogenesis.
- Just as illness is stressful, being depressed is stressful, which triggers a further biochemical cascade of additional stress hormones that deepen the depression. More anxiety and stress produce ever greater depression.
- Depression is linked to chronic inflammation. The increased inflammation from depression reduces neurogenesis even more, which contributes to deepening the depression. Lowering inflammation is now seen as important in fighting depression.

Research into depression is some of the work that led to seeing the importance of neurogenesis and BDNF levels. High levels of neurogenesis and BDNF appear to be mutually exclusive to depression. Additionally, depression is linked not only to reduced neurogenesis but to cognitive decline as well, which is just what we would expect. [34]

Reduced Blood Flow Impairs Our Abilities to Think

In addition to these sources of stress-induced diminishing brain function, stress alters the blood flow in the brain. Stress brings more blood to the lower brain centers concerned with survival while decreasing blood flow to the neocortex and areas responsible for creativity, higher thought, and self-control. **Less blood flow to our higher brain centers means that under stress we literally cannot think as well.** [20]

When we're relaxed and feeling safe, thinking becomes more intuitive, creative, expansive. We see the bigger picture. But under stress, with the exception of a few high performers, we tend to choke and think along stereotypic lines, making hasty, poor decisions that increase stress rather than alleviating it. Stressful thinking leads to more bad decisions that increase stress, leading to worse thinking and more depression. Stress engenders more stress.

And Now for the Really Scary News

What makes this picture really alarming is realizing what causes all this stress. After all, if it was only an occasional lion strolling by every few days or an attack by a neighboring tribe every few years, we could recover and reestablish homeostasis and protect our brains fairly easily. However, what we face is much more daunting.

Remember, it's not just this kind of reptilian brain or limbic system stress that humans experience: it's neocortex-produced psychological stress that is the real problem. **This is the source of chronic stress.**

Daily life is stressful for most people. One poll found 66% of women 18–29 feel "considerable to moderate" stress daily. Worse, 54% said their stress level had increased in the last year. A 2013 poll reported that among millennials, half are so stressed they can't sleep at night, and 39% say their stress levels have increased in the past year. [19]

Our society is stressful and getting more so. Economic uncertainty; work is stressful (and being out of work even more stressful); being unable to control larger forces that affect us; discrimination; the always online culture of being continually plugged in to cell phones, iPads, computers and rarely getting downtime, which creates a faster and faster pace of living—these are some of the easily identified sources of chronic stress. But there are others that can be even more insidious.

Stressful relationships. This includes:

- Bad bosses who are domineering, controlling, lacking empathy, on power trips, or just plain incompetent or mal-attuned
- Bullying relationships
- Hostile or angry relationships
- Personal (non-work) relationships that are emotionally cold or distant, without much personal disclosure
- "As if" relationships that pretend to be more than they are
- Inauthentic relationships
- Anxious relationships
- Being a caretaker
- Codependent relationships
- Relationships with a lot of unexpressed hurt or disappointment
- Abusive relationships

This list could stretch on for many pages, but you get the point. The existential philosopher Jean-Paul Sartre was famously said to have remarked, "Hell is other people." (No wonder he produced such a depressing philosophy.) This "relationship stress" is linked to higher death rates. [36] This daily stress from difficult relationships takes a considerable toll.

Now for the Good News

Before getting too stressed about how stress is killing us, it's important to understand that almost all of this is within our power to control and change. *How we relate to stressful events is key.*

There is tremendous variability in how people deal with stressful situations. Stress can be transformed so that bad stress is replaced by good stress. The chapter "Heart" details ways to transform stress to enhance brain function rather than diminish it.

Poison #3: Physical Assaults

Because of the extreme delicacy and complexity of the brain, it is highly vulnerable to injury from a crash to the head, such as a car accident or fall. Such a blow shakes all the internal "wiring" and jumbles the complex interconnections among neurons. University of California, San Francisco researcher Kristine Yaffe, M.D., presented a study at the Alzheimer's Association International Conference in 2011 that showed a single concussion doubles a person's chances of getting Alzheimer's or other brain diseases later in life. [34]

Protecting the brain from such traumatic shocks is part of good brain hygiene. The chapter "Body" shows how even such everyday activities as running and biking can be done with brain safety in mind.

Physical assaults also come in the form of chemicals and environmental pollution. **Mercury, which accumulates by eating many kinds of fish, is the second most neurotoxic substance**

in the world after plutonium. Even a tiny amount of mercury destroys neurons. Microscopic videos of this process (viewable on YouTube) show neurons shriveling up and dying rapidly at the slightest exposure to a few mercury molecules.

Lead is another environmental pollutant whose levels have now been decreased through EPA guidelines, but not before millions of children and adults had ingested enough lead to permanently lower I.Q.'s and reduce brain function. Children are most at risk for brain damage from substances such as lead and mercury, for in their developing brains the damage can be tenfold compared to adult brains.

Other assaults to the brain include major and minor strokes. Major strokes are often debilitating when they aren't fatal. Far more common are minor, micro-strokes that go unnoticed, but over years they ravage the brain and reduce cognitive capacity.

The High Energy Needs of the Brain

Another source of physical assault on the brain is oxidative damage, which is part of the normal wear and tear that happens continuously. The brain is only 2% of the body by weight but uses 20% of the body's blood flow as well as 20–30% of its energy (oxygen and glucose). The brain needs massive amounts of energy, in the form of glucose, to perform its myriad functions of running our lives and bodies. This high metabolic rate also produces high amounts of free radicals that can damage brain cells if we're low on antioxidant capacity. Strengthening antioxidant capacity through the kind of diet recommended in this book is another way of protecting your neural environment.

Poison #4: Deprivation

When rats are placed in a deprived, impoverished environment where they are understimulated, neurogenesis drops and BDNF levels plunge. What is a deprived environment for a mouse? And, more importantly, what is a deprived environment for human beings?

A tiny cage with only the bare necessities of food and water constitutes a deprived environment for a mouse. No running wheels, no places to explore, no social interaction with other mice, no bright colors or sounds or sensory stimulation, no nesting materials, no change in the daily monotony of living alone with no chance to exercise, interact, explore the world. This is mouse hell. The results are depression, lethargy, neurogenesis practically stops in its tracks, and BDNF levels fall precipitously.

These same effects appear in primates that have been studied. And although human brain studies done on autopsies show very similar results, definitive work is still underway. Nevertheless, the work done so far shows that human brains follow an identical pattern of decline when faced with a deprived, impoverished environment.

When deprivation occurs in infancy or childhood, the results are even more devastating. **Monkeys deprived of maternal care show lifelong anxiety, high stress, social isolation, and lifelong disruptions of brain systems even under new circumstances.**

Children who spent years in low quality orphanages suffered some of this kind of deprivation. They show striking delays in cognitive and social development precisely as animal studies indicate. Autism skyrockets, language development suffers and may never catch up even with remedial work, and brain activity is reduced in key areas, including the hippocampus, amygdala, prefrontal cortex, and brain stem. [21-25]

It is clear that for human beings, a neurally deprived, impoverished environment ravages neurogenesis and brain health. The extreme form of this environment would be solitary confinement in prison. Not only is such an environment bad for the brain, it is emotionally destabilizing for many. While some inmates can survive and stimulate their brains through reading or writing, for many it has long-term negative consequences.

Such an environment is not much different to what many seniors who live alone experience, or patients confined to hospital wards or other institutional care. There is at least a minimal kind of social contact in such situations, but brain stimulation is low, sometimes with only a TV to provide sensory and cognitive stimulation. At least TV can help, but it is no replacement for the real world of other people, nature, and new experiences.

Deprivation can exist at any level of our beings—physical, emotional, mental, spiritual.

- Physical deprivation includes lack of exercise, poor diet, lack of sensory stimulation, color, music, etc.
- Emotional deprivation includes isolation and loneliness as well as interpersonal contact that is strictly superficial, lacking in genuine caring or attachment bonds.
- Mental deprivation means lack of intellectual stimulation, lack of reading, or having conversations about ideas, no opportunity for new learning or exposure to new things.
- Spiritual deprivation consists of starving the soul of its deeper longings for spirit, no participation in a religious or spiritual community, lack of meaning, lack of access to ritual, meditation, or spiritual practices or people.

Deprivation on any of these levels can cause neurogenesis to slow and the brain to wither.

The Brain Thrives on Stimulation

"Use it or lose it" is an adage generally directed to older people who want to age well. However, even in children the brain needs stimulation to develop. And when adulthood is reached, to keep neurogenesis and BDNF levels high, stimulation is essential.

In laboratory studies, mice or monkeys who are placed in an enriched environment show striking increases in neurogenesis and BDNF levels. As mentioned earlier, fewer than half of new brain cells survive to become working parts of our brains. However, when placed in an enriched environment *80–100% of new brain cells survive and integrate into the brain.*

These are some of the effects an enriched environment has on mice, rats, primates, and other mammals:

- increased neurogenesis [26]
- increased synaptogenesis
- an increase in cerebral cortices with 25% more synapses [27,28]
- an increase in the length and complexity of dendrite arbors, which the synapses form upon
- higher order dendrite complexity [29,30]
- increased blood flow to the brain with greater capillary density and width [31,32]
- a boost in brain energy by increasing the volume of neuron mitochondria (which provides energy to the cell) by an astonishing 20% [32]
- an increase in the number of glial cells by 12–14%, an expansion of their cell nuclei by 37.5% [26,32]

These increases in the brain's neurons, blood flow, energy, supporting glial connections, and synapses are breathtaking. If some substance could bring about this amount of brain improvement, it would quickly become the most prized substance in the world. **Yet each of us can bring about these changes in our own brain if we want to.**

The previous five chapters focus on what to do to increase neurogenesis; this chapter shows the equally important need to avoid decreasing neurogenesis.

Future Dreams

In the future the governments of the world will clean up the environment, the oceans, air, and earth. It will be safe to eat any kind of fish without fear of mercury contamination. Civilizations across the globe will value the health of their citizens' brains and invest heavily in education, so every brain will learn as much as it can. Environmental awareness is high, and no one will even try to lobby Congress for higher mercury or lead levels because any corporation would be too ashamed to try to make money at the expense of children's growing brains.

People will eat an anti-inflammatory and anti-oxidant rich diet. Fast food restaurants will switch to healthy alternatives and eliminate fried foods and high sugar meals. Businesses and corporations will provide stress checkups for their employees to make sure no one works too hard or overtaxes their resources. Time off to reset the body's homeostatic balance and lower stress hormones will be a part of everyone's lifestyle.

Summary

This chapter looks at four major poisons to the brain. By knowing what is neurotoxic, you can minimize or avoid altogether what slows down neurogenesis. The main culprits are:

- chronic inflammation
- chronic stress
- physical assaults (brain injury or toxins like mercury or lead)
- deprivation (lack of sensory or mental stimulation, lack of emotional or spiritual connection)

Reducing chronic inflammation and chronic stress are essential to increase neurogenesis and have a healthy brain. It is necessary to protect your brain from physical assaults and not deprive it of the optimal stimulation that feeds it.

CHAPTER 9

PUTTING IT ALL TOGETHER:
TOWARD A NEUROGENIC LIFESTYLE

Enhancing neurogenesis is a lifestyle. A neurogenic diet and lifestyle promotes neurogenesis and minimizes those things that slow it down. To make the most of our lives, we need to make the most of our brains.

The theme of this book is that to increase neurogenesis, your whole being—body, heart, mind, spirit—needs to be aligned with the brain's "project" of bringing forth its potentials. Your brain renews itself by engaging with the world, through developing your skills and talents, your physical abilities, your emotional powers for connection, love, and empathy, by using your mind and awakening your spirit.

This is the path to continuous renewal: ongoing neurogenesis through actualizing our capacities and self. We need to use our entire brains. Brain enhancement equals life enhancement.

Isn't it extraordinary that the growth and health of our brains are the natural results of fully using what we are given? **When we use what we have, we flourish.**

What we don't use withers and falls away, whether it's neurons that are pruned, muscles that atrophy, or skills that get rusty. The good news is that it's never too late. The brain is always changing. Even very late in life there are many things we can do to stimulate neurogenesis and fresh growth.

The sooner we begin a neurohealthy life, the greater the payoff in the long run. Studies are clear that the earlier in life neurogenesis is stimulated, the greater the effect on brain health. The hippocampal area is thicker in enriched animals, showing a greater number of neurons and dendritic connections. Interestingly, even when the enrichment is withdrawn in this case, increased neurogenesis continues. It seems obvious that the earlier we begin a neurogenic lifestyle the greater its impact on our brains and lives.

The sooner we do anything, the more of a developmental influence it will be on body and brain. But as long as we are alive, the brain is renewing itself. Beginning environmental enrichment in middle age results in a fivefold increase in neurogenesis in old age. [1] Thus far there is little research on beginning an enriched environment in old age. Becoming more active by enhancing our brains' renewal in our seventies and eighties yields powerful results. Far better to do something and improve your life going forward than do nothing and decay more rapidly. **As long as we are alive, greater renewal is possible.** The benefits of an "active life" for older adults are clear. Neurogenesis is always happening, and we can always increase its rate. It may seem daunting at first to create a lifestyle to support neurogenesis and brain health. There is so much to do it can seem overwhelming.

Begin with what feels easy. Then let the other steps develop. Start with what you're comfortable with, whether it's taking specific nutrients or beginning to exercise more regularly or get a better night's sleep. Everything helps. For many this is how it begins: taking the first steps toward a neurohealthy lifestyle. **Any step forward toward health is not to be minimized but supported.** One step leads to the next.

Starting with a cafeteria-style approach engenders the least resistance. Doing more of what you already do or beginning activities you already want to try or adding nutrients that are easy to include in your diet are natural starting points. As these changes become habitual and routine, it's less of a stretch to add other activities or nutrients, to experiment with new ways to stimulate your body, heart, mind, or spirit.

To make the most of what's given us in this life means to increasingly harmonize our lives with our brains' possibilities for renewal and neurogenesis. A neurogenic lifestyle stimulates neurogenesis and avoids what slows it down. Remember, it's a two-pronged approach.

A neurogenic lifestyle is something we grow into. It doesn't spring forth fully formed like Zeus from his father's head. It's more like altering the course of an ocean liner. It takes time to shift our habitual patterns and head in a neurohealthy direction. But the more we incline in this direction, the better we feel. The better we feel, the more we're reinforced to feel even better by making more changes.

Start from where you are. If you can't run, then walk, and gradually walk more and faster. If you have a lot of stress in your life, start to reduce it. If you don't sleep much, try to sleep more. Positive change begets more positive change.

Over time, anyone will see that a neurogenic lifestyle feels good. And we naturally want to do more. We don't have to force ourselves or "should" ourselves. When we align with our own deepest natures, we hardly even need to make an effort. Our natural tendencies come forth and carry us on our way in an almost effortless effort. Before we know it we find life more fully aligned with our brain in a neurohealthy lifestyle.

The Good Life

Becoming our highest and best selves involves using our brains' full potentials—physical, emotional, mental, and spiritual. This means exercising our choices in life, and making neurohealthy rather than neurotoxic choices in our daily living.

When we don't actualize our potentials, we feel bad. There is a kind of sickness of the soul that sets in when our deeper selves are frustrated, whether the obstacles are inner or outer. It feels bad when we can't exercise our powers or explore what's possible. When one part of us can't develop, say our minds or our bodies, there is a deep inward disappointment that feels like some part of us is drying up and withering away. Not being able to bring ourselves forth is a pain unlike any other, a sickness of the soul. Although related to depression it goes beyond it. This deep pain may be the pain of neurogenesis slowing down. It's the pain of potential thwarted.

On the other hand, it feels so good when we do allow our selves to come out and play, to become what we can be, to explore what's possible. Neurogenesis accelerates as our physical, emotional, mental, and spiritual sides flourish. When neurogenesis is high, we tend to feel really good. Even when bad things happen, we have much more inner resources to deal with them.

The good news is that what's best for our brains is also what's best for us. Our brains want us to enjoy ourselves, want us to engage with life and become ourselves. By doing what we are made for, we bring forth our greater self and renew ourselves simultaneously.

Expanding our brains means expanding our lives. Finding love, health, happiness, and fulfillment comes by exercising all of who we are. The end of this book is just the beginning…

APPENDIX A.

A BRIEF TOUR OF YOUR BRAIN

Let's take a quick look at some of the brain's most important systems. These are four of the key ways to understand the extraordinary physical-emotional-mental-spiritual consciousness that the brain expresses.

1. The three structures by which the brain has evolved, from the reptilian brain to the mammalian brain to the human brain
2. The right and left hemispheres of the brain that see the world differently and work together
3. The central role of emotion in brain functioning and how it integrates different brain systems to bring coherence to our experience of living
4. The importance of the hippocampus for brain health and optimal function

1. The Triune Brain

The human brain is the masterpiece of evolution. While there are many ways of talking about the brain, one of the most useful was developed by neuroscientist Paul MacLean in his book, *The Triune Brain In Evolution* [1] and later popularized by Carl Sagan.

The evolutionarily oldest part of the brain is the reptilian brain stem, which controls our basic bodily functions and primitive survival circuits. Heart rate, breathing, digestion, sweating, elimination, and the other bodily processes can keep going even if the rest of the brain isn't functioning (such as when someone is declared "brain dead").

The reptilian brain stem's survival circuits contain the "fight-or-flight" response of the autonomic nervous system. Here we have the sympathetic and the parasympathetic systems.

Imagine you're driving along the highway and suddenly a car cuts in front of you and slams on the brakes! You immediately feel a surge of adrenaline and other stress hormones as you react. This is the sympathetic nervous system in action. It gets you going in times of threat or stress. Later on in the safety of your home you can settle down and relax more fully. This is due to the parasympathetic nervous system, which returns us to homeostasis and lets us feel calm, relaxed, and safe.

Together these two systems control arousal and calming. Too much arousal and we're constantly stressed, anxious, hypervigilant, fearful, even leading to panic attacks. Too much calming and we're lethargic, slow, numb. An optimal balance is ideal.

While the reptilian brain stem is the first to develop in the womb, the next development in evolution was the mammalian brain, or limbic system. **The limbic system brings forth emotion**

and bonding. Mammals bond with their young. Reptiles do not and some even eat their young.

Mice, rats, horses, elephants, lions, humans, and other mammals all share a common limbic system that allows us to feel an emotional connection to others—other people as well as other mammals. Gazing into the warm eyes of an elephant or deer or dog creates an emotional connection that transcends form.

The limbic system picks up on and greatly expands the survival circuits of the reptilian brain stem. The reptilian brain's stress response of "fight or flight" enlists the limbic system to amplify its reactions, and a structure known as the amygdala is called into action especially when fear or anger are triggered. It is key in all emotional learning. As we'll see shortly, emotion has great significance for how the brain works. The limbic system is the second brain system to develop in utero.

The third brain system is evolution's newest development and the last to develop in utero: the neocortex. **The neocortex is the source of language, abstract thought, and most of what we think of as "human."** The neocortex gives us language, music, science, history and culture. It allows one generation to learn from the previous generation and build upon it.

The large size of the neocortex is what sets humans apart from all other mammals. In humans the neocortex is 30% of the brain. In dogs the neocortex is 7% of the brain. In cats it's 3%. Chimpanzees have 11% of their brains for the neocortex. [3] Birds have no neocortex, which is why calling someone a "birdbrain" is an insult. The neocortex gives us the greatest attainments of human civilization. It is evolution's supreme achievement.

The crown jewel of the neocortex is called the prefrontal cortex. Some have even called the prefrontal cortex a "fourth brain," since it brings forth the highest achievements humans are capable of. It is responsible for creativity, empathy, insight, morality, and executive function, which is our capacity to plan, to regulate our emotions, to postpone immediate gratification for the sake of future goals. The prefrontal cortex develops after birth. [2]

Three Brains in One

These three "brains" are stacked on top of each other to form layers of the brain. The human brain consists of a vertical integration of these three brain systems.

Each of these brains has evolved to overcome the limitations of the previous brain, while incorporating the information the earlier brain provides. The neocortex, especially the prefrontal cortex, is the integrator and director of these three brains.

Full brain development requires a safe and nurturing environment. The size and quality of an infant's brain depends upon the mother's emotional state. When a pregnant woman feels nourished and safe, she will give birth to a baby that has an enlarged neocortex and a small reptilian brain stem. **This safety during pregnancy allows for ideal brain growth so the higher brain systems can unfold.**

However, when the expectant mother is anxious, isolated, or stressed, she gives birth to a baby with an enlarged reptilian brain and a reduced neocortex. It's as if fear switches on the survival circuits and shuts down everything else. Nature must first ensure survival before developing the brain's higher capacities. Such a child starts life with a neural disadvantage, less capacity to plan, to control impulses, to be thoughtful and creative.

The mother's emotional state continues to have a dramatic effect on the baby's brain development for several years after birth as well. Children with mothers who are stressed, anxious, traumatized, or depressed show diminished prefrontal cortex development and greater reptilian survival-circuit brains. [2] Later development can compensate for these early developmental deficits, but since 90% of brain growth happens during the first two years of life, just how much can be overcome is at present unknown. [5]

Optimal brain development gives us access to our animal inheritance—the reptilian survival circuits and the mammalian capacity for emotion—together with our reason and intelligence.

The Arc of Development

As these three brains develop across the lifespan, there are advantages and disadvantages to each stage of development. Childhood is concerned with the initial growth and working together of these three brains. The neocortex, especially the prefrontal cortex, isn't fully formed until the early twenties. That's why adolescents tend to be so impulsive—they simply don't have the full brain structure by which their impulses can be modulated and regulated.

It's only in our early twenties that we have a fully developed brain. But brain development doesn't stop there. It continues until we die.

Young mature brains of those in their twenties and thirties have fast processing speed and better working memory. Our capacities to learn new facts quickly is at its height, as well as our abilities to process and deal with new information of great complexity. Problem solving in novel situations is high. Reflexes are fast. There is rapid adaptability to new environments,

However, these young brains also have some drawbacks. There is greater hemispheric specialization, which means that younger brains rely more heavily on one side of the brain or the other. There is a tendency to "shoot from the hip" without knowing all the facts. Perception is more egocentric and less able to take in the viewpoints of others than later in life.

Mature brains of people in their fifties, sixties, seventies, and beyond have their own strengths. Rather than simply being a decline of once good brain function, **aging confers greater capacities upon the brain, while also reducing some other abilities.** There is more accumulated knowledge, so crystallized intelligence tends to rise. There is greater integration between the right and left sides of the brain, which gives both a better perspective of the whole as well as of the part.

Additionally, mature brains are better at emotion regulation and so are less impulsive and less reactive to negative emotions from others. They are driven less by dopamine (a reward neurotransmitter that underlies much of the pleasure of sex, drugs, and gambling). Older people are able to integrate multiple perspectives, which allows for better abilities to compromise and empathically understand the other. Understanding of interpersonal complexity is greater.

Part of the wisdom from aging comes from greater myelination in two areas of the brain: the frontal lobes and temporal lobes. Greater myelination (which peaks around age fifty and in some cases age sixty) means greater coating of neurons that allows them to fire more efficiently and faster. These two areas of the brain are responsible for decision-making, emotion regulation, language, and memory. [9, 10]

In short, we want our fighter pilots to be in their twenties and thirties, while we want the President and decision makers to have mature brains that develop after forty or fifty.

It is important to note, however, the enormous differences in how brains age. Some brains age exceedingly well and are as sharp as a tack into their nineties and past a hundred. **Wisdom can deepen as long as we are alive.**

Other brains fare poorly and show signs of decline in the late thirties or forties. Others decline more gradually but still unnecessarily in their fifties, sixties, and seventies. Brains exposed to toxic environments, poor diets, lack of exercise, little mental stimulation, and interpersonal isolation show rapid deterioration. [7] There is much more likelihood of cognitive decline, dementia, and Alzheimer's when more of these factors are present.

Taking Responsibility for Our Self-Changing Brains

What is so remarkable about the brain is that it changes through its own actions. That is, the brain makes decisions about what it will be exposed to: what foods to eat, what people to be around, what work to do, what exercise to do (or not). **The brain creates its own future by the choices it makes in the present.**

Without knowledge, our choices are bound to be unskillful, even though we may be doing the best we can. But with knowledge we can choose to create a brain-healthy life that will upgrade our brains to keep them vital, alive, and feeling good throughout our lifespans. Your brain has its destiny in its own hands. This book is a road map.

2. Right and Left Hemispheres

In many respects the two hemispheres of the brain work in similar ways. Yet they also process information in different, complementary ways. The right hemisphere (which controls the left side of the body) is:

- visuospatial
- musical
- works in intuitive leaps
- has an integrated map of the whole body
- is primarily responsible for the stress response
- holds our autobiographical memory
- allows us to feel empathy

The left brain (which controls the right side of the body), on the other hand is:

- verbal
- analytical
- logical
- linear
- allows for abstract thinking
- can divorce thought from feeling
- is the dominant hemisphere for most people

The right brain listens to the music while the left brain hears the words.

Our brains integrates both these modes of processing to produce our experiences. Both sides are necessary for producing a complete picture of the world and our inner experiences.

We can see the whole (right brain) as well as slice the whole into smaller and smaller parts to better understand the world (left brain). We can empathize with what another person is feeling (right brain) and share with the person through language that we know how it feels (left brain). We can feel our feelings (right brain) and know what we are feeling by reflecting on it and naming it (left brain). We can experience something (right brain) and we can stand back and observe it by being self-reflective (left brain). We need both sides of our brains to give us a complete picture of our inner and outer worlds.

True, certain tasks may rely on one side more than the other. A musician develops the right hemisphere more while an accountant develops the left. But most jobs and most things in life require both sides of our brains.

Over the centuries, literacy and science have produced a left hemisphere–dominant culture. But as computers and images play a greater role in daily life, the right hemisphere is currently getting new emphasis. Perhaps we are moving toward a more balanced brain culture in the future.

3. Emotion organizes the brain

Neuroscientists stress how crucial emotion is for organizing the many different streams of information coming into the brain. [4, 6] Out of the huge amount of information streaming into the brain—thoughts, sensations, memories, desires—we need some way to make sense of it. Feeling does this—quickly and without logical thinking.

Emotion coordinates our experiences so we understand the world. Feelings integrate many streams of neural processing—thinking, sensing, impulse, motivation, and action. The result is a smooth, cohesive functioning that guides our activities and choices.

Our feelings tell us *what* to pay attention to, *how* to pay attention to it, and they *evaluate* what we pay attention to. Further, our feelings tell us what to do and motivate us to do it.

Our every voluntary act has a feeling behind it, even if we aren't aware of what it is. This is why in severe depression where feeling has been replaced with dead numbness, the person can't even get out of bed—there is no feeling to motivate it. When we numb our feelings, we deaden ourselves. **We are alive to the extent that we can feel.**

Recent research has revolutionized our ideas about emotion. We now know it is much more pervasive than previously thought.

Emotion is our guide in life. Thinking only tells us so much about the world and other people. We need feeling to guide us toward or away from people and situations.

There are eight universal emotions common to every culture in the world, which emotion research and cross-cultural studies have confirmed. [11] Three of these feelings (listed in their lower and higher intensities) are positive:

- caring/love
- interest/excitement
- enjoyment/joy
- Five of these feelings are negative:
- fear/terror
- anger/rage
- sadness/depression
- embarrassment/shame
- disgust

Of course even the "negative" emotions are positive in that they are evolutionarily adaptive; "negative" simply means they feel bad.

We need to discern which feelings to act on and which to definitely not act on. **In a perfect world we would learn to really listen to our hearts' emotional guidance. This would lead us** to people who love us for our authentic selves, toward work that is intrinsically interesting and joyful, and activities that bring joy and happiness. We would spend most of our lives in the three positive emotions. These positive feelings, when they're fairly continuous, increase neurogenesis, immunity, and cognitive function.

But this world is far from perfect. In the real world, we don't fully listen to our hearts' guidance. Since everyone on this planet is wounded in growing up and learns to push away certain feelings, this leads to painful relationships, alienating work, and a mood characterized by negative feelings of anxiety, stress, fear, anger, depression, and shame. **When these negative feelings become chronic, neurogenesis decreases significantly, cognitive function declines, and the brain shrinks.**

4. The Importance of the Hippocampus for Brain Function

Like many brain systems, there is a hippocampus on the right and left sides of the brain that are mirror images of each other. Technically we have two hippocampi, although it is usually referred to in the singular. The hippocampus has two ends, the temporal (or ventral) and the septal (or dorsal). The temporal end connects to areas of the brain involved in emotion and how the brain regulates feelings. The septal end is most involved in memory, new learning, and cognition. This side connects to other brain systems that mediate body awareness and spatial processing as well as thinking and learning (body and mind).

The hippocampus processes new memories, aggregates their different data streams, and then organizes them to provide a feeling of continuity through time. The hippocampus doesn't store new memories but creates them. A well-documented case study illustrates how critical the hippocampus is in forming new memories.

The case of "Mr. Underwood" was presented in *A General Theory of Love* as a man with a brain injury that destroyed his hippocampus. He always believed it was 1985 and that Ronald Reagan was president. His doctors and nurses would introduce themselves to him every day, and for him it was the first time he'd met them. He'd tell the same jokes three or four times within 10–15 minutes. He had access to his old memories, for these were stored elsewhere in the brain. But because his hippocampus was gone, he was stuck in the present moment without having continuity with the past. [8]

The hippocampus allows new memories to form. Alzheimer's and other neurodegenerative diseases that attack the hippocampus interfere with making new memories. Old established memories are often accessible, but forming new memories is disrupted. **This capacity to form new memories and to place situations in context requires a healthy hippocampus.** We understand where we are and what's going on as the hippocampus continues to aggregate different strands of experience and integrate this into our ongoing stream of memory. Without this capacity, we're lost, as so many Alzheimer's patients are.

The temporal end of the hippocampus is involved in emotion regulation. It appears that particularly stress regulation and depression regulation are affected by the hippocampus. Lower rates of neurogenesis in this portion of the hippocampus make a person vulnerable to depression and the debilitating effects of chronic stress. High rates of neurogenesis in the temporal end, on the other hand, are protective against stress, anxiety, fear, and depression. [13]

High levels of stress hormones, such as glucocorticoids, have a toxic effect on hippocampal neurons. In fact, high glucocorticoid levels can kill neurons in the hippocampus. Since the ability to modulate stress hormones is one function of the hippocampus, the more stress spirals out of control, the more damage to the stress-regulating systems of the hippocampus is done, which lessens the person's ability to regulate stress and the neurotoxic stress hormones. A negative spiral ensues: rising stress hormones, lower rates of neurogenesis, and impaired ability to regulate stress, which further raises glucocorticoid levels and further damages and reduces the brain's ability to turn off the toxic stream. [12]

Meditation, prayer, and devotional spiritual practices increase the size of the hippocampus along its entire length. The level of spirit appears to be strongly impacted by hippocampal functioning.

It's clear that the hippocampus is central to all four levels of our consciousness: body, heart, mind, spirit. It may be the most essential part of our brains, the key to our identities and lives.

How the Brain Grows

What stimulates neurogenesis and neural growth are various chemical messengers known as neurotrophins. These include: nerve growth factor (NGF), which is involved in sympathetic and sensory neurons; neurotrophin-3 (NT-3), which is involved in sensory neurons; the less well studied neurotrophin-4 (NT-4); and the much studied brain-derived neurotrophic factor (BDNF). *BDNF has received a great deal of attention because it is so prominent in adult neurogenesis and those brain systems related to memory, learning, and cognition.* It is now seen to be central in recovery from depression and stress as well.

BDNF: Your New Best Friend

Brain-derived neurotrophic factor—it's quite a mouthful. Let's stick with the acronym BDNF.

BDNF is the main signal that "turns on" neurogenesis and stimulates neural plasticity. BDNF, along with other neurotrophins, allows the brain to grow. Neural growth includes neurogenesis, neurite outgrowth (axon or dendrite growth), synaptogenesis, and the development of dendritic spines. Remember, ongoing new growth and pruning of old growth happens simultaneously.

The constant flow of information to the brain means that connections between neurons are in a continuous process of strengthening and weakening, depending on use. With repetition connections get stronger ("Neurons that fire together wire together"). With lack of use connections are pruned.

An enriched environment increases BDNF levels in the brain, stimulating neurogenesis and neural growth. A stressful or impoverished environment (including chronic stress, anxiety, fear, and depression) decreases BDNF levels and dramatically inhibits neurogenesis and brain development.

Birth and Survival

Brain health depends not only on new brain cells forming but surviving. In normal neurogenesis about 60–70% of new neurons die off. However, in a highly enriched environment almost all new neurons survive. Thus, our hope for optimal brain vitality is both to increase the rate of neurogenesis *and* to increase the survival rate for these new brain cells.

BDNF is important for both

As mentioned earlier, artificially increasing BDNF levels in the brain by injecting it into the organism had the opposite effect than was expected. It interfered with cognition and memory and neurogenesis. There is an incredible network of safety mechanisms in the brain that cannot simply be overridden.

This oversimplifying of the brain's complexity was the error behind the "serotonin deficiency" theory of depression. Big Pharma's attempt to cure depression by artificially increasing one of the more than twenty neurotransmitters involved in mood is sometimes compared with trying to do brain surgery with a blunt axe. Even when it does work, it may do so along entirely different lines than what was anticipated and in the process can do violence to the brain's interconnected, complex protective systems and throw off its homeostatic balance.

Trying to bypass the brain's natural processes is playing with fire. As a clinical psychologist I find it truly scary when I see the hubris displayed in experimenting with powerful, mind-altering drugs. Granted, sometimes this medication is helpful and necessary, but they are now prescribed so readily and with such a cavalier attitude that I see many people who are numbed, medicated, overstimulated or artificially bubbly, and only "half there."

One way to see the current spate of zombie movies is as an expression of the culture's collective consciousness about overmedication turning so many people into numbed zombies. The lack of humility before the brain's incalculable complexity gives me pause. We experiment like this at our own peril.

We don't want to trick the brain; we want to work with the brain.

Summary

This appendix highlights the main systems of the brain, including its triune structure:

- the reptilian brain stem that runs most of the body's systems
- the mammalian limbic system, or emotional brain
- the highly developed neocortex responsible for language and abstract thinking

The left and right hemispheres of the brain are explained, along with how emotion is central in organizing the brain.

The hippocampus gets special emphasis, for this structure is intertwined with every level of our being: body, heart, mind, spirit. As the main area where neurogenesis occurs, the hippocampus processes new memories, which gives us our sense of continuity in time and space. Without this we are lost.

Finally, BDNF is a key neurotrophin that stimulates neurogenesis. Working with the brain to increase neurogenesis and BDNF levels respects the brain's protective systems rather than trying to override them with an artificial drug.

GLOSSARY

amygdala: The part of the brain that detects fear, prepares for emergency events and gives an immediate emotional appraisal of events.

amyloid plaques: A starchlike protein-carbohydrate complex deposited in brain tissue, it is one of the two brain abnormalities that constitute Alzheimer's disease, the other being neurofibrillary tangles.

axon: The part of a nerve cell that conducts a nerve impulse from one cell to another via a synapse.

beta-amyloid, also called amyloid-beta: The key protein in the amyloid plaques found in Alzheimer's disease.

BDNF: Brain-derived neurotrophic factor is a kind of "miracle grow" for the brain that stimulates neurogenesis and synaptogenesis as well as promotes neuron survival.

biomarkers: Biological markers or indicators of certain biological processes.

BMP: Bone morphogenetic protein consists of a family of growth factors that promote the formation of bone and the skeleton, as well as help mend broken bones.

catechins: A type of antioxidant compound or flavanol found in tea, and in lesser amounts in red wine, chocolate, and apples.

caloric restriction (CR): A diet that has all the required nutrients but with less calories than are usually consumed.

cognitive function: This is the mental process of knowing, including aspects such as awareness, perception, reasoning, feeling, and judgment.

cognitive reserve: This indicates both the resilience of a brain as well as the extra resources that can be used for neural processing (e.g., memory, thinking), different mental pathways utilized to reach an intellectual goal.

cytokines: These are a category of proteins that send signals between cells and have an inflammatory effect.

daidzein: An isoflavone or compound found primarily in soybeans and some other legumes.

dendrite: The branching, root-like ending of a nerve cell that receives impulses from other cells.

depth psychology: The understanding that humans have an unconscious aspect, beyond their conscious thinking, feeling, and sensing.

excitotoxicity: The damage or killing of nerve cells due to excessive stimulation.

flavonoids: Also known as bioflavonoids, flavonoids are plant compounds that are antioxidants and occur as pigments in fruit and flowers.

free radicals (ROS): Free radicals (or reactive oxygen species) are unstable molecules that have at least one unpaired electron and are therefore capable of rapid chain reactions that destabilize other molecules. They can be very damaging to body tissue and are one of the key elements of aging.

genistein: A phytoestrogen (similar to estrogen) that is an isoflavone found especially in soybeans.

glial cells: These are the most abundant cells in the central nervous system. They are non-neural cells that perform housekeeping functions such as cleaning out debris and accumulated toxins, protecting, and pruning the brain.

glucocorticoids: Steroid hormones (such as hydrocortisone) that are released during stress.

glycation: The bonding of a sugar molecule to a protein or fat resulting in damage or destruction of the tissue. It is associated with increased oxidative damage and is a major component of aging.

glymphatic system: The brain's system for cleaning itself is a functional waste-clearance pathway of cerebrospinal fluid that flushes out accumulated toxins and amyloid-beta, primarily at night during sleep.

hippocampus: The part of the brain involved in forming new memories, it also plays a critical role in reasoning and remembering as well as emotion regulation and spatial memory. Damage to the hippocampus results in cognitive deficits and memory problems.

intersectionality: Human individuality is multifaceted, and some categories of our identity may be oppressed while others may be privileged, for we live in many worlds simultaneously.

isoflavones: These comprise a class of compounds found in many legumes, but primarily in soybeans, that act as estrogens in mammals and are antioxidants.

insulin resistance: When the body is overwhelmed with more sugar than it can handle, the cells make fewer insulin receptors. This diminishes the ability of cells to respond to insulin, and is often a precursor to type 2 diabetes.

LDL molecules: Low-density lipoprotein was long considered "the bad cholesterol," but new research shows it consists of two main subtypes: large, "fluffy" molecules that are not harmful, and very low-density small molecules that do significant damage to the cardiovascular system. Special blood tests are required to make this differentiation.

limbic system: The limbic system is the emotional brain in humans and other mammals.

macrophages: These specialized white blood cells protect the body from infection and ingest foreign particles.

mild cognitive impairment (MCI): Mild cognitive impairment is the intermediate stage between the expected decline of normal aging and the more serious decline of dementia.

neocortex: The neocortex is the most recent evolutionary development in mammalian brains and is most advanced in humans. It is responsible for humans' capacity for abstract reasoning, language, creativity, and self-awareness.

neural plasticity: This allows the brain to make new connections among neurons and to heal, to some degree, after traumatic brain injuries or strokes.

neurodegenerative diseases: These are diseases that affect the brain and central nervous system, such as Alzheimer's, Parkinson's, and multiple sclerosis (MS).

neurogenesis: This is the process of creating new neurons, or brain cells.

neuron: A neuron is a brain cell.

neuroscience: A branch of science focused on studying the brain.

neurotrophins: These are a class of growth factors that help in the production, survival, development, and function of neurons or brain cells.

NGF: Nerve growth factor, one of the neurotrophins.

omega-3 fatty acids: These essential fats are anti-inflammatory, antioxidant, stimulate neurogenesis, and must be consumed in the diet.

omega-6 fatty acids: These are essential (must be taken in through diet) but inflammatory and problematic when consumed in too large amounts. (The typical Western diet has far too much omega-6 and needs more omega-3s to counterbalance their effects.)

oxidation (free radical damage): Like rust or the browning of a newly cut apple, oxidation is an interaction between oxygen molecules and different substances, ranging from metal to living tissue. A key element of aging, antioxidants from the diet and formed within the body protect from the degenerative effects of oxidation.

oxytocin: A hormone and neurotransmitter involved in love, trust, empathy, pro-social behavior, and feeling good.

polyphenols: These antioxidants are phenolic compounds found in many fresh fruits and vegetables.

prefrontal cortex: This is the most recent evolutionary development in the human brain, the part responsible for our highest capacities, such as creativity, executive function, empathy, science, and religion.

PTSD: Post-traumatic stress disorder.

selective serotonin reuptake inhibitors (SSRIs): A class of antidepressants that selectively block the brain from reabsorbing the neurotransmitter serotonin after it has been released.

serotonin: A neurotransmitter involved in mood, sleep, and appetite. Ninety percent of the body's serotonin is located in the intestinal tract, where it regulates intestinal movements.

synapse: The synapse is the gap between brain cells, where information flows between neurons by way of an electro-chemical signal.

synaptogenesis: The process of growing new synapses or connections between neurons.

tau: Tau is a protein that helps stabilize neural structures in healthy brains, but when damaged (hyperphosphorylation), it can create the tangles involved in Alzheimer's disease.

trans fats: The most dangerous type of fat, they cannot be metabolized by the body and damage the blood vessels, heart, brain, and other organs.

REFERENCES

Upgrade Your Brain and Upgrade Your Life

1. Gage, F. (2011). "Interview with the Science Network." (12/11/2011) online.

2. Gage, F. (1998). "Neurogenesis in the adult human hippocampus." *Nature Medicine.* 4, 1313–1317.

3. Santarelli, L. (2003). "Requirement of hippocampal neurogenesis for the behavioral effects of antidepressants." *Science.* 301(5634):805–809. doi: 10.1126/science.1083328.

4. Malberg, J. E., Eisch, A. J., Nestler, E. J., & Duman, R. S. (2000). "Chronic antidepressant treatment increases neurogenesis in adult rat hippocampus." *The Journal of Neuroscience: The official journal of the Society for Neuroscience.* 20(24):9104–10. PMID: 11124987.

5. Gage, F. (Aug 2000). "Reinventing the brain." *Life Extension Magazine* interview.

6. Tanapat, P., Galea, L., Gould, E. (1998). "Stress inhibits the proliferation of granule cell precursors in the developing dental gyrate." *International Journal of Developmental Neuroscience.* 16:235–9.

7. Sapolsky, R. (1999). "Stress and your shrinking brain." *Discover.* 20(3):116–122.

8. Gould, E., Tanapat, P. (1 Dec 1999). "Stress and hippocampal neurogenesis." *Biological Psychiatry.* 46(11):1472–9.

9. Kubera, M., Obuchowicz, E., Goehler L., Brzeszcz J., Maes, M. (Aug 2010). "In animal models, psychosocial stress-induced

(neuro)inflammation, apoptosis and reduced neurogenesis are associated to the onset of depression." *Progress in Neuro-Psychopharmacology and Biological Psychiatry.*

10. Kempermann, G., Kuhn, H. G., Gage, F. H. (Apr 1997). "More hippocampal neurons in adult mice living in an enriched environment." *Nature.* 3:386(6624):493–5.

11. (Aug 2002). "Neuroplasticity in old age: Sustained fivefold induction of hippocampal neurogenesis by long-term environmental enrichment." *Annals of Neurology.* 52(2):135–43.

12. Kempermann, G., Gast, D., Gage, F. H. (Oct 2013). "Cell tissue res." 354(1):203–19. doi: 10.1007/s00441-013-1612-z. Epub 18 Apr 2013.

13. Tanti, A., Belzung, C. "Hippocampal neurogenesis: A biomarker for depression or antidepressant effects? Methodological considerations and perspectives for future research."

14. Kempermann, G., Kuhn, G., Gage, F. (1 May 1998). "Experience-induced neurogenesis and the senescent dentate gyrus." *Journal of Neuroscience.* 18(9):3206–3212.

The Program

1. Gage, F. (2011). "Interview with the Science Network." (12/11/2011) online.

Diet

1. Casadesus, G., Shukitt-Hale, B., Stellwagen, H. M., et al. (Oct 2004). "Modulation of hippocampal plasticity and cognitive behavior by short-term blueberry supplementation in aged rats." *Nutritional Neuroscience.* 7(5–6):309–16.

2. Acosta, S., Jernberg, J., Sanberg, C. D., Sanberg, P. R., Small, B. J., Gemma, C., Bickford, P. C. (Oct 2010). Rejuvenation Res. 13(5):581–8. doi: 10.1089/rej.2009.1011. Epub 29 Jun 2010.

3. Joseph, J. A., Shukitt-Hale, B., Lau, F. C. "Fruit polyphenols and their effects on neuronal signaling and behavior in senescence." *Annals of the New York Academy of Sciences.*

4. Joseph, J. A., Denisova, N. A., Arendash, G., et al. (June 2003). "Blueberry supplementation enhances signaling and prevents behavioral deficits in an Alzheimer disease model." *Nutritional Neuroscience.* 6(3):153–62.

5. Joseph, J. A., Carey, A., Brewer, G. J., Lau, F. C., Fisher, D. R. (July 2007). "Dopamine and abeta-induced stress signaling and decrements in Ca2+ buffering in primary neonatal hippocampal cells are antagonized by blueberry extract." *Journal of Alzheimer's Disease.* 11(4):433–46.

6. Devore, E. E., Kang, J. H., Breteler, M. M., Grodstein, F. A. (July 2012). "Dietary intakes of berries and flavonoids in relation to cognitive decline." *Neurology.* 72(1):135–43. doi: 10.1002/ana.23594. Epub 26 Apr 2012.

7. Joseph, J. A., Shukitt-Hale, B., Willis, L. M. (Sep 2009). "Grape juice, berries, and walnuts affect brain aging and behavior." *Journal of Nutrition.* 139(9):1813S–7S. doi: 10.3945/jn.109.108266. Epub 29 Jul 2009. Review.

8. Dai, Q., Borenstein, A. R., Wu, Y., Jackson, J. C., Larson, E.B. (Sep 2006). "Fruit and vegetable juices and Alzheimer's disease: The kame project." *American Journal of Medicine.* 119(9):751–9.

9. Lau, F. C., Shukitt-Hale, B., Joseph, J. A. (2007). "Nutritional intervention in brain aging: Reducing the effects of inflammation and oxidative stress." *Subcell Biochemistry.* 42:299–318.

10. McGeer, P. L., McGeer, E. G. (May 2004). "Inflammation and neurodegeneration in Parkinson's disease." *Parkinsonism Related Disorders.* 10 Suppl 1:S3–S7.

11. Joseph, J. A., Denisova, N. A., Arendash, G., et al. (June 2003). "Blueberry supplementation enhances signaling and prevents behavioral deficits in an Alzheimer disease model." *Nutritional Neuroscience.* 6(3):153–62.

12. Joseph, J. A., Carey, A., Brewer, G. J., Lau, F. C., Fisher, D. R. (July 2007). "Dopamine and abeta-induced stress signaling and decrements in Ca2+ buffering in primary neonatal hippocampal cells are antagonized by blueberry extract." *Journal of Alzheimer's Disease.* 11(4):433–46.

13. Shukitt-Hale, B., Carey, A. N., Jenkins, D., Rabin, B. M., Joseph, J. A. (Aug 2007). "Beneficial effects of fruit extracts on neuronal function and behavior in a rodent model of accelerated aging." *Neurobiological Aging.* 28(8):1187–94.

14. McGuire, S. O., Sortwell, C. E., Shukitt-Hale, B., et al. (Oct 2006). "Dietary supplementation with blueberry extract improves survival of transplanted dopamine neurons." *Nutritional Neuroscience.* 9(5-6):251–8.

15. Suh, N., Paul, S., Hao, X., et al. (1 Jan 2007). "Pterostilbene, an active constituent of blueberries, suppresses aberrant crypt foci formation in the azoxymethane-induced colon carcinogenesis model in rats." *Clinical Cancer Research.* 13(1):350–5.

16. Heinonen, M. (June 2007). "Antioxidant activity and antimicrobial effect of berry phenolics—a Finnish perspective." *Molecular Nutrition and Food Research.* 51(6):684–91.

17. Russell, W. R., Labat, A., Scobbie, L., Duncan, S.H. (June 2007). "Availability of blueberry phenolics for microbial metabolism in the colon and the potential inflammatory implications." *Molecular Nutrition and Food Research.* 51(6):726–31.

18. Zafra-Stone, S., Yasmin, T., Bagchi, M., et al. (June 2007). "Berry anthocyanins as novel antioxidants in human health and disease prevention." *Molecular Nutrition and Food Research.* 51(6):675–83.

19. (26 Mar 2007). *Neuroscience Letters.* 415(2):154–158. Epub 7 January 2007. doi: 10.1016/j.neulet.2007.01.010. PMCID: PMC1892224. NIHMSID: NIHMS20377.

20. Beltz, B. S., Tlusty, M. F., Benton, J. L., and Sandeman, D. C. "Omega-3 fatty acids upregulate adult neurogenesis."

21. Conklin, S. M., Gianaros, P. J., Brown, S. M., et al. (29 June 2007). "Long-chain omega-3 fatty acid intake is associated positively with corticolimbic gray matter volume in healthy adults." *Neuroscience Letters.* 421(3):209–12.

22. Wurtman, R. J., Cansev, M., Sakamoto, T., Ulus, I. H. (2009). "Use of phosphatide precursors to promote synaptogenesis." *Annual Review of Nutrition.* 29:59–87.

23. Wurtman, R. J., Cansev, M., Ulus, I. H. (Mar 2009). "Synapse formation is enhanced by oral administration of uridine and DHA, the circulating precursors of brain phosphatides." *Journal of Nutrition Health and Aging*. 13(3):189–97.

24. Heinrichs, S. C. (Apr 2010). "Dietary omega-3 fatty acid supplementation for optimizing neuronal structure and function." *Molecular Nutrition & Food Research*. 54(4):447–56.

25. Hibbeln, J. (2001). "Interview with Life Extension magazine October report."

26. Jockers, D. (2012). "Is your brain getting enough of this nutrient?" *NaturalNews.com*. (11/05/2012).

27. Beltz, B. S., Tlusty, M. F., Benton, J. L., Sandeman, D. C. (2007). "Omega-3 fatty acids upregulate adult neurogenesis." *Neuroscience Letters*.

28. Freemantle, E., Vandal, M., Tremblay-Mercier, J., Tremblay, S., Blachere, J. C., Begin, M. E., Brenna, J. T., Windust, A., Cunnane, S. C. (2006). "Omega-3 fatty acids, energy substrates, and brain function during aging." *Prostaglandins Leukotrienes and Essential Fatty Acids*. 75:213–220.

29. Gomez-Pinilla, F. (2008). "Brain foods: The effects of nutrients on brain function." *Nature Reviews Neuroscience*. 9:568–578.

30. (Aug 2012). *Molecular Nutrition & Food Research*. 56(8):1292–303. doi: 10.1002/mnfr.201200035. Epub 13 Jun 2012.

31. Wang, Y., Li, M., Xu, X., Song, M., Tao, H., Bai, Y. "Green tea epigallocatechin-3-gallate (EGCG) promotes neural progenitor cell proliferation and sonic hedgehog pathway activation during adult hippocampal neurogenesis."

32. Goepp, J. (Apr 2008). "New research on the benefits of green tea." *Life Extension*.

33. Yoo, K. Y., Choi, J. H., Hwang, I. K., Lee, C. H., Lee, S. O., Han, S. M., Shin, H. C., Kang, I. J., Won, M. H. (July 2010). "Epigallocatechin-3-gallate increases cell proliferation and neuroblasts in the subgranular zone of the dentate gyrus in adult mice." *Phytotherapy Research*. 24(7):1065–70. doi: 10.1002/ptr.3083.

34. Han, M. E., Park, K. H., Baek, S. Y., Kim, B. S., Kim, J. B., Kim, H. J., Oh, S. O. (18 May 2007). "Inhibitory effects of caffeine on hippocampal neurogenesis and function." *Biochemical and Biophysical Research Communications.* 356(4):976–80. Epub 26 Mar 2007.

35. Wentz, C. T., Magavi, S. S. (May–June 2009). "Caffeine alters proliferation of neuronal precursors in the adult hippocampus." *Neuropharmacology.* 56(6–7):994–1000. doi: 10.1016/j. neuropharm.2009.02.002. PMID: 19217915. Epub 13 Feb 2009.

36. Kim, S. J., Son, T. G., Park, H. R., Park, M., Kim, M. S., Kim, H. S., Chung, H. Y., Mattson, M. P., Lee, J. (23 May 2008). "Curcumin stimulates proliferation of embryonic neural progenitor cells and neurogenesis in the adult hippocampus." *Journal of Biological Chemistry.* 283(21):14497–505. doi: 10.1074/jbc.M708373200. Epub 24 Mar 2008.

37. Ng, T. P., Chiam, P. C., Lee, T., Chua, H. C., Lim, L., Kua, E. H. (1 Nov 2006). "Curry consumption and cognitive function in the elderly." *American Journal of Epidemiology.* 164(9):898–906. Epub 26 Jul 2006.

38. Bhutani, M. K., Bishnoi, M., Kulkarni, S. K. (Mar 2009). "Antidepressant like effect of curcumin and its combination with piperine in unpredictable chronic stress-induced behavioral, biochemical and neurochemical changes." *Pharmacology Biochemistry and Behavior.* 92(1):39–43. doi: 10.1016/j. pbb.2008.10.007. Epub 25 Oct 2008.

39. Singh, N., Bhalla, M., de Jager, P., Gilca, M. (2011). "An overview on ashwagandha: A Rasayana (rejuvenator) of Ayurveda." *African Journal of Traditional Complementary and Alternative Medicine.* 8(5 Suppl):208–13. doi: 10.4314/ajtcam. v8i5S.9. Epub 3 July 2011.

40. Singh, N., Bhalla, M., de Jager, P., Gilca M. (2011). "An overview on ashwagandha: A rasayana (rejuvenator) of Ayurveda." *African Journal of Traditional Complementary and Alternative Medicine.* 8(5 suppl):208–13. doi: 10.4314/ajtcam. v8i5S.9. Epub 3 Jul 2011.

41. Gupta, G. L., Rana, A. C. (Oct–Dec 2007). "Protective effect of Withania somnifera dunal root extract against protracted social

isolation induced behavior in rats." *Indian Journal of Physiology and Pharmacology.* 51(4):345–53.

42. Rivera, P., Pérez-Martín, M., Pavón, F. J., Serrano, A., Crespillo, A., Cifuentes, M., López-Ávalos, M. D., Grondona, J. M., Vida, M., Fernández-Llebrez, P., de Fonseca, F. R., Suárez, J. (31May 2013). "Pharmacological administration of the isoflavone daidzein enhances cell proliferation and reduces high fat diet-induced apoptosis and gliosis in the rat hippocampus." *PLoS One.* 8(5):e64750. doi: 10.1371/journal. pone.0064750.

43. Zheng, J., Zhang, P., Li, X., Lei, S., Li, W., He, X., Zhang, J., Wang, N., Qi, C., Chen, X., Lu, H., Liu, Y. (12 Feb 2013). "Post-stroke estradiol treatment enhances neurogenesis in the subventricular zone of rats after permanent focal cerebral ischemia." *Neuroscience.* 231:82–90. doi: 10.1016/j. neuroscience.2012.11.042. Epub 2 Dec 2012.

44. Bayer, J., Rune, G., Kutsche, K., Schwarze, U., Kalisch, R., Büchel, C., Sommer, T. (Feb 2013). "Estrogen and the male hippocampus: Genetic variation in the aromatase gene predicting serum estrogen is associated with hippocampal gray matter volume in men." *Hippocampus.* (2):117–21. doi: 10.1002/ hipo.22059. Epub 6 Aug 2012.

45. Barha, C. K., Galea, L. A. (Mar 2013). "The hormone therapy, Premarin, impairs hippocampus-dependent spatial learning and memory and reduces activation of new granule neurons in response to memory in female rats." *Neurobiology of Aging.* 34(3):986–1004. doi: 10.1016/j.neurobiolaging.2012.07.009. Epub 28 Aug 2012.

46. Okamoto, M., Hojo, Y., Inoue, K., Matsui, T., Kawato, S., McEwen, B. S., Soya, H. (7 Aug 2012). "Mild exercise increases dihydrotestosterone in hippocampus providing evidence for androgenic mediation of neurogenesis." *Proceedings of the National Academy of Science USA.* 109(32):131005. doi: 10.1073/ pnas.1210023109. Epub 17 Jul 2012.

47. Hall, Z. J., Macdougall-Shackleton, S. A. (2012). "Influence of testosterone metabolites on song-control system neuroplasticity during photostimulation in adult European starlings (Sturnus

vulgaris)." *PLoS One.* 7(7):e40060. doi: 10.1371/journal. pone.0040060. Epub 6 Jul 2012.

48. Barker, J. M., Ball, G. F., Balthazart, J. (7 Nov 2013). "Anatomically discrete sex differences and enhancement by testosterone of cell proliferation in the telencephalic ventricle zone of the adult canary brain." *Journal of Chemical Neuroanatomy.* doi: pii: S0891–0618(13)00089-6. 10.1016/j. jchemneu.2013.10.005.

49. Spritzer, M. D., Ibler, E., Inglis, W., Curtis, M. G. (10 Nov 2011). "Testosterone and social isolation influence adult neurogenesis in the dentate gyrus of male rats." *Neuroscience.* 195:180–90. doi: 10.1016/j.neuroscience.2011.08.034. Epub 19 Aug 2011.

50. Lee, C. H., Kim, J. M., Kim, D. H., Park, S. J., Liu, X., Cai, M., Hong, J. G., Park, J. H., Ryu, J. H. (Sep 2013). "Effects of sun ginseng on memory enhancement and hippocampal neurogenesis." *Phytotherapy Research.* 27(9):1293-9. doi: 10.1002/ptr.4873. Epub 29 Oct 2012.

51. Lin, T., Liu, Y., Shi, M., Liu, X., Li, L., Liu, Y., Zhao, G. (1 Aug 2012). "Promotive effect of ginsenoside Rd on proliferation of neural stem cells in vivo and in vitro." *Journal Ethnopharmacology.* 142(3):754–61. doi: 10.1016/j. jep.2012.05.057. Epub 7 Jun 2012.

52. Jiang, B., Xiong, Z., Yang, J., Wang, W., Wang, Y., Hu, Z. L., Wang, F., Chen, J. G. (July 2012). "Antidepressant-like effects of ginsenoside Rg1 are due to activation of the BDNF signalling pathway and neurogenesis in the hippocampus." *British Journal of Pharmacology.* 166(6):1872–87. doi: 10.1111/j.1476-5381.2012.01902.x.

53. Zheng, G. Q., Cheng, W., Wang, Y., Wang, X. M., Zhao, S. Z., Zhou, Y., Liu, S. J., Wang, X. T. (27 Jan 2011). "Ginseng total saponins enhance neurogenesis after focal cerebral ischemia." *Journal of Ethnopharmacology.* 133(2):724–8. doi: 10.1016/j. jep.2010.01.064. Epub 10 Nov 2010.

54. Zainuddin, M. S. A., & Thuret, S. (2012). "Nutrition, adult hippocampal neurogenesis and mental health." *British Medical Bulletin.* 103, 1, p. 89–114. DOI:10.1093/bmb/lds021."

55. Scholey, A., Owen, L. (Oct 2013). "Effects of chocolate on cognitive function and mood: A systematic review." *Nutrition Review.* 71(10):665–81. doi: 10.1111/nure.12065.

56. Sokolov, A. N., Pavlova, M. A., Klosterhalfen, S., Enck, P. (26 June 2013). "Chocolate and the brain: Neurobiological impact of cocoa flavanols on cognition and behavior." *Neuroscience & Biobehavioral Reviews.* pii: S0149–7634(13)00168–1. doi: 10.1016/j.neubiorev.2013.06.013.

57. Tchantchou, F., Lacor, P. N., Cao, Z., Lao, L., Hou, Y., Cui, C., Klein, W. L., Luo, Y. (2009). "Stimulation of neurogenesis and synaptogenesis by bilobalide and quercetin via common final pathway in hippocampal neurons." *Journal of Alzheimer's Disease.* 18(4):787–98. doi: 10.3233/JAD-2009-1189.

58. Yoo, D. Y., Nam, Y., Kim, W., Yoo, K. Y., Park, J., Lee, C. H., Choi, J. H., Yoon, Y. S., Kim, D. W., Won, M. H., Hwang, I. K. (Jan 2011). "Effects of Ginkgo biloba extract on promotion of neurogenesis in the hippocampal dentate gyrus in C57BL/6 mice." *Journal of Veterinary Medical Science.* 73(1):71–6. Epub 30 Aug 2010.

59. Zainuddin, M. S. A. & Thuret, S. (2012). "Nutrition, adult hippocampal neurogenesis and mental health." *British Medical Bulletin.* 103 (1) 89–114. doi: 10.1093/bmb/lds021.

60. Park, H. R., Kong, K. H., Yu, B. P., Mattson, M. P., Lee, J. (14 Dec 2012). "Resveratrol inhibits the proliferation of neural progenitor cells and hippocampal neurogenesis." *Journal of Biological Chemistry.* 287(51):42588–600. doi: 10.1074/jbc. M112.406413. Epub 26 Oct 2012.

61. Moriya, J., Chen, R., Yamakawa, J., Sasaki, K., Ishigaki, Y., Takahashi, T. (2011). "Resveratrol improves hippocampal atrophy in chronic fatigue mice by enhancing neurogenesis and inhibiting apoptosis of granular cells." *Biological and Pharmaceutical Bulletin.* 34(3):354–9.

62. Wang, J., Gallagher, D., DeVito, L. M., Cancino, G. I., Tsui, D., He, L. Keller, G. M., Frankland, P. W., Kaplan, D. R., Miller, F. D. (6 July 2012). "Metformin activates an atypical PKC-CBP pathway to promote neurogenesis and enhance spatial memory formation." *Cell Stem Cell.* 11(1): 23–35.

63. Funakoshi, H., Kanai, M., and Nakamura, T. (2011). "Modulation of tryptophan metabolism, promotion of neurogenesis and alteration of anxiety-related behavior in tryptophan 2,3-dioxygenase-deficient mice." *International Journal of Tryptophan Research.* 4:7–18. Epub 11 Apr 2011. doi: 10.4137/IJTR.S5783. PMCID: PMC3195223.

64. Qu, Z., Zhou, Y., Zeng, Y.,* Lin, Y., Li, Y., Zhong, Z., and Chan, W. Y., (2012). "Protective effects of a Rhodiola crenulata extract and salidroside on hippocampal neurogenesis against streptozotocin-induced neural injury in the rat." *PLoS One.* 7(1):e29641. doi: 10.1371/journal.pone.0029641. PMCID: PMC3250459. Epub 3 Jan 2012.

65. Fiorentini, A., Rosi, M. C., Grossi, C., Luccarini, I., Casamenti, F. (2010). "Lithium improves hippocampal neurogenesis, neuropathology and cognitive functions in APP mutant mice." *PLoS One.* 5(12):e14382. doi: 10.1371/journal.pone.0014382. Epub 20 Dec 2010.

66. Sarlak, G., Jenwitheesuk, A., Chetsawang, B., Govitrapong, P. (20 Sep 2013). "Effects of melatonin on nervous system aging: Neurogenesis and neurodegeneration." *Journal of Pharmacological Sciences.* 123(1):9–24. Epub 27 Aug 2013.

67. Ramírez-Rodríguez, G., Vega-Rivera, N. M., Benítez-King. G., Castro-García, M., Ortíz-López, L. (14 Nov 2012). "Melatonin supplementation delays the decline of adult hippocampal neurogenesis during normal aging of mice." *Neuroscience Letters.* 530(1):53–8. doi: 10.1016/j.neulet.2012.09.045. Epub 6 Oct 2012.

68. Chern, C. M., Liao, J. F., Wang, Y. H., Shen, Y. C. (1 May 2012). "Melatonin ameliorates neural function by promoting endogenous neurogenesis through the MT2 melatonin receptor in ischemic-stroke mice." *Free Radical Biology & Medicine.* 52(9):1634–47. doi: 10.1016/j.freeradbiomed.2012.01.030. Epub 10 Feb 2012.

69. Kim, H. G., Oh, M. S. (14 July 2013). "Memory-enhancing effect of Mori Fructus via induction of nerve growth factor." *British Journal of Nutrition.* 110(1):86–94. doi: 10.1017/S0007114512004710. Epub 27 Nov 2012.

70. Zhuang, P., Zhang, Y.,* Cui, G., Bian, Y., Zhang, M., Zhang, J., Liu, Y., Yang, X., Isaiah, A. O., Lin, Y., and Jiang, Y. (2012). "Direct stimulation of adult neural stem/progenitor cells in vitro and neurogenesis in vivo by salvianolic acid B." *PLoS One.* 7(4):e35636. doi: 10.1371/journal.pone.0035636 PMCID: PMC3335811. Epub 24 Apr 2012.

71. Lau, B. W., Lee, J. C., Li, Y., Fung, S. M., Sang, Y. H., Shen, J., Chang, R. C., So, K. F. (2012). "Polysaccharides from wolfberry prevents corticosterone-induced inhibition of sexual behavior and increases neurogenesis." *PLoS One.* 7(4):e33374. doi: 10.1371/journal.pone.0033374. Epub 16 Apr 2012.

72. Kondziella, D., Strandberg, J., Lindquist, C., Asztely. F. (26 Jan 2011). "Lamotrigine increases the number of BrdU-labeled cells in the rat hippocampus." *NeuroReport.* 22(2):97–100. doi: 10.1097/WNR.0b013e328342d2fa.

73. Yoo, D. Y., Kim, W., Yoo, K. Y., Lee, C. H., Choi, J. H., Yoon, Y. S., Kim, D. W., Won, M. H., Hwang, I. K. (May 2011). "Grape seed extract enhances neurogenesis in the hippocampal dentate gyrus in C57BL/6 mice." *Phytotherapy Research.* 25(5):668–74. doi: 10.1002/ptr.3319. Epub 29 Oct 2010.

74. Yang, W. M., Shim, K. J., Choi, M. J., Park, S. Y., Choi, B. J., Chang, M. S., Park, S. K. (3 Oct 2008). "Novel effects of Nelumbo nucifera rhizome extract on memory and neurogenesis in the dentate gyrus of the rat hippocampus." *Neuroscience Letters.* 443(2):104–7. doi: 10.1016/j. neulet.2008.07.020. Epub 11 Jul 2008.

75. Wen, J., Yang, B. N., Ren, D. Zhongguo Zhong Xi Yi Jie He Za Zhi. (Mar 2010). "Effect of Lycium barbarum polysaccharides on neurogenesis and learning & amp: Memory in manganese poisoning mice." 30(3):295–8. Chinese.

76. Miao, Y., Ren, J., Jiang, L., Liu, J., Jiang, B., Zhang, X. (Nov 2013). "α-lipoic acid attenuates obesity-associated hippocampal neuroinflammation and increases the levels of brain-derived neurotrophic factor in ovariectomized rats fed a high-fat diet." *International Journal of Molecular Medicine.* 32(5):1179–86. doi: 10.3892/ijmm.2013.1482. Epub 5 Sep 2013.

77. Cimini, A., Gentile, R., D'Angelo, B., Benedetti, E., Cristiano, L., Avantaggiati, M. L., Giordano, A., Ferri, C., Desideri, G. (Oct 2013). "Cocoa powder triggers neuroprotective and preventive effects in a human Alzheimer's disease model by modulating BDNF signaling pathway." *Journal of Cellular Biochemistry.* 114(10):2209–20. doi: 10.1002/jcb.24548.

78. Abumaria, N., Yin, B., Zhang, L., Li, X. Y., Chen, T., Descalzi, G., Zhao, L., Ahn, M., Luo, L., Ran, C., Zhuo, M., and Liu, G. (19 Oct 2011). "Effects of elevation of brain magnesium on fear conditioning, fear extinction, and synaptic plasticity in the infralimbic prefrontal cortex and lateral amygdala." *Journal of Neuroscience.* 31(42):14871–14881. doi: 10.1523/JNEUROSCI.3782-11.2011.

79. Liu, G. (2012). "Prevention of cognitive deficits in Alzheimer's mouse model by elevating brain magnesium." *Molecular Neurodegeneration.* 7(suppl 1):L24. doi: 10.1186/1750-1326-7-S1-L24. Epub 7 Feb 2012.

80. Leyhe, T., Eschweiler, G. W., Stransky, E., Gasser, T., Annas, P., Basun, H., Laske, C. (2009). "Increase of BDNF serum concentration in lithium treated patients with early Alzheimer's disease." *Journal of Alzheimer's Disease.* 16(3):649–56. doi: 10.3233/JAD-2009-1004.

81. Hashimoto, R., Takei, N., Shimazu, K., Christ, L., Lu, B., Chuang, D. M. (Dec 2002). "Lithium induces brain-derived neurotrophic factor and activates TrkB in rodent cortical neurons: An essential step for neuroprotection against glutamate excitotoxicity." *Neuropharmacology.* 43(7):1173–9.

82. Corona, C., Frazzini, V., Silvestri, E., Lattanzio, R., La Sorda, R., Piantelli, M., Canzoniero, L. M. T., Ciavardelli, D., Rizzarelli, E., Sensi, S. L. (2011). "Effects of dietary supplementation of carnosine on mitochondrial dysfunction, amyloid pathology, and cognitive deficits in 3xTg-AD mice." *PLoS One.* 6(3):e17971. doi: 10.1371/journal.pone.0017971. Epub 15 March 2011.

83. Murakami, T., Furuse, M. (July 2010). "The impact of taurine- and beta-alanine-supplemented diets on behavioral and neurochemical parameters in mice: Antidepressant

versus anxiolytic-like effects." *Amino Acids.* 39(2):427–34. doi: 10.1007/s00726-009-0458-x. Epub 23 Jan 2010.

84. Kiraly, S. J., Kiraly, M. A., Hawe, R. D., and Makhani, N. (2006). "Vitamin D as a neuroactive substance: Review." *Scientific World Journal.* 6:125–139.

85. Li, L. F., Lu, J., Li, X. M., Xu, C. L., Deng, J. M., Qu, R., Ma, S. P. (Aug 2012). "Antidepressant-like effect of magnolol on BDNF up-regulation and serotonergic system activity in unpredictable chronic mild stress treated rats." *Phytotherapy Research.* 26(8):1189–94. doi: 10.1002/ptr.3706. Epub 5 Jan 2012.

86. Li, S., Wang, C., Wang, M., Li, W., Matsumoto, K., Tang, Y. (20 Mar 2007). "Antidepressant like effects of piperine in chronic mild stress treated mice and its possible mechanisms." *Life Science.* 80(15):1373–81. Epub 12 Jan 2007.

87. Kittur, S., Wilasrusmee, S., Pedersen, W. A., Mattson, M. P., Straube-West, K., Wilasrusmee, C., Lubelt, B., Kittur, D. S. (June 2002). "Neurotrophic and neuroprotective effects of milk thistle (Silybum marianum) on neurons in culture." *Journal of Molecular Neuroscience.* 18(3):265–9.

88. Tsai, S. J. (2006). "Cysteamine-related agents could be potential antidepressants through increasing central BDNF levels." *Medical Hypotheses.* 67(5):1185–8. Epub Jun 22, 2006.

89. Moriguchi, S., Shinoda, Y., Yamamoto, Y., Sasaki, Y., Miyajima, K., Tagashira, H., Fukunaga, K. (8 Apr 2013). "Stimulation of the sigma-1 receptor by DHEA enhances synaptic efficacy and neurogenesis in the hippocampal dentate gyrus of olfactory bulbectomized mice." *PLoS One.* 8(4):e60863. doi: 10.1371/journal.pone.0060863.

90. (July 2006). "Therapeutic potential of neurogenesis for prevention and recovery from Alzheimer's disease: Allopregnanolone as a proof of concept neurogenic agent." *Current Alzheimer's Research.* 3(3):185–90.

91. (Apr 2006). "Effects of huperzine A on memory deficits and neurotrophic factors production after transient cerebral ischemia and reperfusion in mice." *Pharmacology Biochemistry and Behavior.* 83(4):603–11. Epub 9 May 2006.

92. Lu, B., Nagappan, G., Xiaoming, G., Pradeep J. N., & Wren, P. (2013). "BDNF-based synaptic repair as a disease-modifying strategy for neurodegenerative diseases." *Nature Reviews Neuroscience.* 14:401–416. doi: 10.1038/nrn3505.

93. Hou, Y., Aboukhatwa, M. A., Lei, D., Manaye, K., Khan, I., and Luo, Y.* (May 2010). "Antidepressant natural flavonols modulate BDNF and beta amyloid in neurons and hippocampus of double TgAD mice." *Neuropharmacology.* 58(6): 911–920. doi: 10.1016/j.neuropharm.2009.11.002. Epub 14 Nov 2009.

94. Molendijk, M. L.,* Haffmans, J. P. M., Bus, B. A. A., Spinhoven, P., Penninx, B. W. J. H., Prickaerts, J., Richard C. Oude Voshaar, R. C., and Elzinga, B. M. (2012). "Serum BDNF concentrations show strong seasonal variation and correlations with the amount of ambient sunlight." *PLoS One.* 7(11): e48046. doi: 10.1371/journal.pone.0048046. PMCID: PMC3487856. Epub 2 Nov 2012.

95. Elzinga, B. M., Molendijk, M. L., Oude Voshaar, R. C., Bus, B. A. A., Prickaerts, J., Spinhoven, P., Penninx, B. J. W. H. (Mar 2011). "The impact of childhood abuse and recent stress on serum brain-derived neurotrophic factor and the moderating role of BDNF Val66Met." *Psychopharmacology* (Berl) 214(1):319–328. Epub 12 August 2010. doi: 10.1007/s00213-010-1961-1.

96. Crupi, R., Mazzon, E., Marino, A., La Spada, G., Bramanti, P., Battaglia, F., Cuzzocrea, S., and Spina, E. (2011). "Hypericum perforatum treatment: Effect on behaviour and neurogenesis in a chronic stress model in mice." *BMC Complementary and Alternative Medicine.* 11:7. doi: 10.1186/1472-6882-11-7. PMCID: PMC3041724. Epub 27 Jan 2011.

97. Jang, S., Dilger, R. N., and Johnson, R. W.* (Oct 2010). "Luteolin inhibits microglia and alters hippocampal-dependent spatial working memory in aged mice1,2,3." *Journal of Nutrition.* 140(10):1892–1898. doi: 10.3945/jn.110.123273. PMCID: PMC2937579. Epub 4 Aug 2010.

98. , M. L.,* Bus, B. A. A., Spinhoven, P., Penninx, B. W. J. H., G., Prickaerts, J., Oude Voshaar, R. C., and Elzinga, B. M. (Nov 2011). "Serum levels of brain-derived neurotrophic

factor in major depressive disorder: State–trait issues, clinical features and pharmacological treatment." *Molecular Psychiatry.* 16(11):1088–1095. doi: 10.1038/mp.2010.98. PMCID: PMC3220395. Epub 21 Sep 2010.

99. Taupin, P. (May 2009). "Apigenin and related compounds stimulate adult neurogenesis." Mars, Inc., the Salk Institute for Biological Studies: WO2008147483. Dublin City University, School of Biotechnology, Glasnevin, Dublin 9, Ireland. Expert Opinion on Therapeutic Patents (Impact Factor: 3.53). 19(4):523–7. doi: 10.1517/13543770902721279.

100. Crupi, R., Paterniti, I., Ahmad, A., Campolo, M., Esposito, E., Cuzzocrea, S. (Nov 2013). "Effects of palmitoylethanolamide and luteolin in an animal model of anxiety/depression." *CNS & Neurological Disorders—Drug Targets.* 12(7):989–1001.

101. Park, H. J., Shim, H. S., Kim, K. S., Han, J. J., Kim, J. S., Ram Yu, A., Shim, I. (Mar 2013). "Enhanced learning and memory of normal young rats by repeated oral administration of krill phosphatidylserine." *Nutritional Neuroscience.* 16(2):47–53. doi: 10.1179/1476830512Y.0000000029. Epub 8 Aug 2012.

102. Maggioni, M., Picotti, G. B., Bondiolotti, G. P., Panerai, A., Cenacchi, T., Nobile, P., Brambilla, F. (Mar 1990). "Effects of phosphatidylserine therapy in geriatric patients with depressive disorders." *Acta Psychiatrica Scandinavica.* 81(3):265–70.

103. Xu, S. L., Bi, C. W. C., Choi, R. C. Y., Zhu, K. Y., Miernisha, A., Dong, T. T. X., and Tsim, K. W. K. (2013). "Flavonoids induce the synthesis and secretion of neurotrophic factors in cultured rat astrocytes: A signaling response mediated by estrogen receptor." *Evidence-Based Complementary and Alternative Medicine Volume 2013.* Article ID 127075. http://dx.doi.org/10.1155/2013/127075.

104. Jin, K., Xie, L., Mao, X. O., Greenberg, D. A. (26 Apr 2006). "Alzheimer's disease drugs promote neurogenesis." *Brain Research.* 1085(1):183–188.

105. Jana, A., Modi, K. K., Roy, A., Anderson, J. A., van Breemen, R. B., Pahan, K. (June 2013). "Up-regulation of neurotrophic factors by cinnamon and its metabolite sodium benzoate: Therapeutic implications for neurodegenerative disorders."

Journal of Neuroimmune Pharmacology. 8(3):739–55. doi: 10.1007/s11481-013-9447-7. Epub 9 Mar 2013.

106. Casadesus, G., Shukitt-Hale, B., Stellwagen, H. M., Zhu, X., Lee, H. G., Smith, M. A., & Joseph, J. A. (2004). "Modulation of hippocampal plasticity and cognitive behavior by short-term blueberry supplementation in aged rats." *Nutritional Neuroscience.* 7:309–316.

107. Sen, C. K., Rink, C., Khanna, S. (June 2010). "Palm oil-derived natural vitamin E alpha-tocotrienol in brain health and disease." *Journal of the American College of Nutrition.* 29(3 Suppl):314S–323S.

108. Kikuchi, S., Shinpo, K., Takeuchi, M., Yamagishi, S., Makita, Z., Sasaki, N., Tashiro, K. (Mar 2003). "Glycation—A sweet tempter for neuronal death." *Brain Research Reviews.* 41(2–3):306–23.

109. van der Borght, K., Köhnke, R., Göransson, N., Deierborg, T., Brundin, P., Erlanson-Albertsson, C., Lindqvist, A. (25 Feb 2011). "Reduced neurogenesis in the rat hippocampus following high fructose consumption." *Regulatory Peptides.* 167(1):26–30. doi: 10.1016/j.regpep.2010.11.002. Epub 27 Nov 2010.

110. Mortby, M. E., Janke, A. L., Anstey, K. J., Sachdev, P. S., Cherbuin, N. (4 Sep 2013). "High 'normal' blood glucose is associated with decreased brain volume and cognitive performance in the 60s: The PATH through life study." *PLoS One.* 8(9):e73697. doi: 10.1371/journal.pone.0073697.

111. Park, H. R., Lee, J. (July 2011). "Neurogenic contributions made by dietary regulation to hippocampal neurogenesis." *Annals for the New York Academy of Sciences.* 1229:23–8. doi: 10.1111/j.1749-6632.2011.06089.x.

112. Park, H. R., Park, M., Choi, J., Park, K. Y., Chung, H. Y., Lee J. (4 Oct 2010). "A high-fat diet impairs neurogenesis: Involvement of lipid peroxidation and brain-derived neurotrophic factor." *Neuroscience Letters.* 482(3):235–9. doi: 10.1016/j.neulet.2010.07.046. Epub 27 Jul 2010.

113. Amen, D. (2012). *Use your brain to change your age.* Crown Archetype: New York.

114. Tozuka, Y., Wada, E., Wada, K. (June 2009). "Diet-induced obesity in female mice leads to peroxidized lipid accumulations and impairment of hippocampal neurogenesis during the early life of their offspring." *FASEB Journal.* 23(6):1920-34. doi: 10.1096/fj.08-124784. Epub 21 Jan 2009.

115. Anderson, M. L., Nokia, M. S., Govindaraju, K. P., Shors, T. J. (8 Nov 2012). "Moderate drinking? Alcohol consumption significantly decreases neurogenesis in the adult hippocampus." *Neuroscience.* 224:202–9. doi: 10.1016/j. neuroscience.2012.08.018. Epub 18 Aug 2012.

116. Briones, T. L., Woods, J. (19 Dec 2013). "Chronic binge-like alcohol consumption in adolescence causes depression-like symptoms possibly mediated by the effects of BDNF on neurogenesis." *Neuroscience.* 254:324–34. doi: 10.1016/j. neuroscience.2013.09.031. Epub 25 Sep 2013.

117. Ehlers, C. L., Liu, W., Wills, D. N., Crews, F. T. (6 Aug 2013). "Periadolescent ethanol vapor exposure persistently reduces measures of hippocampal neurogenesis that are associated with behavioral outcomes in adulthood." *Neuroscience.* 244:1–15. doi: 10.1016/j.neuroscience.2013.03.058. Epub 6 Apr 2013.

118. Wentz, C. T., Magavi, S. S. (May-Jun 2009). "Caffeine alters proliferation of neuronal precursors in the adult hippocampus." *Neuropharmacology.* 56(6–7):994–1000. doi: 10.1016/j. neuropharm.2009.02.002. Epub 13 Feb 2009.

119. Han, M. E., Park, K. H., Baek, S. Y., Kim, B. S., Kim, J. B., Kim, H. J., Oh, S. O. (18 May 2007). "Inhibitory effects of caffeine on hippocampal neurogenesis and function." *Biochemical and Biophysical Research Communications.* 356(4):976–80. Epub 26 Mar 2007.

120. Akazawa, Y., Kitamura, T., Fujihara, Y., Yoshimura, Y., Mitome, M., Hasegawa, T. (Feb 2013). "Forced mastication increases survival of adult neural stem cells in the hippocampal dentate gyrus." *International Journal of Molecular Medicine.* 31(2):307–14. doi: 10.3892/ijmm.2012.1217. Epub 18 Dec 2012.

121. Yamamoto, T., Hirayama, A., Hosoe, N., Furube, M., Hirano, S. (Aug 2009). "Soft-diet feeding inhibits adult neurogenesis

in hippocampus of mice." *Bulletin of Tokyo Dental College.* 50(3):117–24.

122. Aoki, H., Kimoto, K., Hori, N., Toyoda, M. (Nov-Dec 2005). "Cell proliferation in the dentate gyrus of rat hippocampus is inhibited by soft diet feeding." *Gerontology.* 51(6):369–74.

123. Patten, A. R., Moller, D. J., Graham, J., Gil-Mohapel, J., Christie, B. R. (19 Dec 2013). "Liquid diets reduce cell proliferation but not neurogenesis in the adult rat hippocampus." *Neuroscience.* 254:173–84. doi: 10.1016/j. neuroscience.2013.09.024. Epub 20 Sep 2013.

124. Zafra-Stone, S., Yasmin, T., Bagchi, M., et al. (June 2012). "Berry anthocyanins as novel antioxidants in human health and disease prevention." *International Journal of Developmental Neuroscience.* 30(4):303–313.

125. Osher, Y., Belmaker, R. H. (Summer 2009). "Omega-3 fatty acids in depression: A review of three studies." *CNS Neuroscience & Therapeutics.* 15(2):128–33.

126.

127. Grayson, D. et al. (5 Feb 2014). "Dietary omega-3 fatty acids modulate large-scale systems organization in the rhesus macaque brain." *Journal of Neuroscience.* 34(6): 2065–2074.

128. (9 Feb 2014). "Fish oil cited in dramatic healing after severe brain trauma." Mercola.com.

129. Arden, J. (2014). *The brain bible.* New York: McGraw-Hill Education.

130. Perlmutter, D. (2013). *Grain brain.* New York: Little, Brown and Company.

131. Nones, J., Leite de Sampaio, S., Gomes, F. (June 2012). "Effects of the flavonoid hesperidin in cerebral progenitors in rats: Indirect action through astrocytes." *International Journal of Developmental Neuroscience.* 30(4) 303–313.

132. Zafra-Stone, S., Yasmin, T., Bagchi, M., et al. (June 2007). "Berry anthocyanins as novel antioxidants in human health and disease prevention." *Molecular Nutrition & Food Research.* 51(6):675–83.

133. Masterjohn, C. (2014). "Learning, your memory, and cholesterol." www.cholesterol-and-health.com.

134. Chowdury, R., et al. (18 March 2014). *Annals of Internal Medicine.*

135. Elias, P., et al. (2005). "Serum cholesterol and cognitive performance in the Framingham heart study." *Psychosomatic Medicine.* 67(1):24–30.

136. West, R., et al. (Sep 2008). "Better memory functioning associated with higher total and low-density lipoprotein cholesterol levels in very elderly subjects without the apolipoprotein e4 allele." *American Journal of Geriatric Psychiatry.* 16(9):998–1002.

137. de la Monte, S., & Wands, J. (Nov 2008). "Alzheimer's disease is type 3 diabetes–evidence reviewed." *Journal of Diabetes Science and Technology.* 2(6):1101–1113.

138. Duckett, S. K., et al. (5 June 2009). "Effects of winter stocker growth rate and finishing system on: III. Tissue proximate, fatty acid, vitamin and cholesterol content" *Journal of Animal Science.* doi: 10.2527/jas 2009-1850.

139. Yaffe, K., Weston, A. L., Blackwell, T., Krueger, K. A. (Mar 2009). "The metabolic syndrome and development of cognitive impairment among older women." *Archives of Neurology.* 66(3):324–8. doi: 10. 1001/archneurol. 2008.566.

140. Reger, M., et al. (Mar 2004). "Effects of beta-hydroxybutryrate on cognition in memory-impaired adults." *Neurobiology of Aging.* 25(3): 311–314.

141. Phivilay, A., et al. (3 Mar 2009). "High dietary consumption of trans fatty acids decreases brain docosahexaenoic acid but does not alter amyloid-beta and tau pathologies in the 3xTg-AD model of Alzheimer's disease." *Neuroscience.* 159(1):296–307.

142. Raji, C., et al. (July 29, 2014). *American Journal of Preventive Medicine.*

143. (July 2011). "Circulation." *Heart Failure Journal.* 4(4):404–413.

144. (August 21, 2014). "Vitamin D for depression, dementia, and diabetes." Mercola.com.

145. Borgwardt, S., Hammann, F., Scheffler, K., Kreuter, M., Drewe, J., Beglinger, C. (Nov 2012). "Neural effects of green tea extract

on dorsolateral prefrontal cortex. *European Journal of Clinical Nutrition.* 66(11):1187–92.

146. Ramírez-Rodríguez, G., Klempin, F., Babu, H., Benítez-King, G., Kempermann, G. (Aug 2009). "Melatonin modulates cell survival of new neurons in the hippocampus of adult mice." *Neuropsychopharmacology.* 34(9):2180–91. doi: 10.1038/npp.2009.46. Epub 6 May 2009.

147. Nones, J., et al. (June 2012). *International Journal of Developmental Neuroscience.* 30(4):303313. doi: 10.1016/i.ijdevneu.2012.01.008

148. Sen, C. K., Khanna, S., Roy, S. (27 Mar 2006). "Tocotrienols: Vitamin E beyond tocopherols." *Life Sciences.* 78(18):2088–98. Epub 3 Feb 2006.

149. Kummerow, F., Kummerow, J. (2014). *Cholesterol is not the culprit.* Spacedoc Media, LLC.

Body

1. Kempermann, G., Gage, F. H. (1999). "Experience-dependent regulation of adult hippocampal neurogenesis: Effects of long-term stimulation and stimulus withdrawal." *Hippocampus.* 9(3):321–32.

2. Leuner, B., Glasper, E. R., Gould, E. (2010) "Sexual experience promotes adult neurogenesis in the hippocampus despite an initial elevation in stress hormones." *PLoS One.* 5(7):e11597. doi:10.1371/journal.pone.0011597.

3. Kempermann, G., Brandon, E. P., Gage, F. H. (30 Jul-13 Aug 1998). "Environmental stimulation of 129/SvJ mice causes increased cell proliferation and neurogenesis in the adult dentate gyrus." *Current Biology.* 8(16):939–42.

4. van Praag, H., Kempermann, G., & Gage, F. H. (1999). "Running increases cell proliferation and neurogenesis in the adult mouse dentate gyrus." *Nature Neuroscience.* 2(266–270). doi: 10.1038/6368.

5. Klaus, F., Amrein, I. (14 Feb 2012). "Running in laboratory and wild rodents: Differences in context sensitivity and plasticity

of hippocampal neurogenesis." *Behavoural Brain Research.* 227(2):363–70. doi: 10.1016/j.bbr.2011.04.027. Epub 27 Apr 2011.

6. van Praag, H. (2008). "Neurogenesis and exercise: Past and future directions." *NeuroMolecular Medicine.* 10(2):128–40. doi: 10.1007/s12017-008-8028-z. Epub 20 Feb 2008.

7. Shechter, R., Baruch, K., Schwartz, M., Rolls, A. (Mar 2011). "Touch gives new life: Mechanosensation modulates spinal cord adult neurogenesis." *Molecular Psychiatry.* 16(3):342–52. doi: 10.1038/mp.2010.116. Epub 16 Nov 2010.

8. Mak, G. K., Antle, M. C., Dyck, R. H., & Weiss, S. (2013). "Bi-parental care contributes to sexually dimorphic neural cell genesis in the adult mammalian brain." *PLoS One*, 8(5):e62701. doi: 10.1371/journal.pone.0062701.

9. Mueller, A. D., Pollock, M. S., Lieblich, S. E., Epp, J. R., Galea, L. A., Mistlberger, R. E. (May 2008). "Sleep deprivation can inhibit adult hippocampal neurogenesis independent of adrenal stress hormones." *American Journal of Physiology: Regulatory Integrative and Comparative Physiology.* 294(5):R1693–703. doi: 10.1152/ajpregu.00858.2007. Epub 20 Feb 2008.

10. Hairston, I. L., Little, M. T. M., Scanlon, M. D., Barakat, M. T., Palmer, T. D., Sapolsky, R. M., and Heller, H. C. (Dec 2005). "Sleep restriction suppresses neurogenesis induced by hippocampus-dependent learning." *American Journal of Psychiatry: Journal of Neurophysiology.* 94(6):4224–4233.

11. Ramirez-Rodriguez, G., Ortíz-López, L., Domínguez-Alonso, A., Benítez-King, G. A., Kempermann, G. (Jan 2011). "Chronic treatment with melatonin stimulates dendrite maturation and complexity in adult hippocampal neurogenesis of mice." *Journal of Pineal Research.* 50(1):29–37.

12. Kim, C. H., Lee, S. C., Shin, J. W., Chung, K. J., Lee, S. H., Shin, M. S., Baek, S. B., Sung, Y. H., Kim, C. J., Kim, K. H. (Sep 2013). "Exposure to music and noise during pregnancy influences neurogenesis and thickness in motor and somatosensory cortex of rat pups." *International Neurourology Journal.* 17(3):107–13. doi: 10.5213/inj.2013.17.3.107. Epub 30 Sep 2013.

13. Kirste, I., Nicola, Z., Kronenberg, G., Walker, T. L., Liu, R. C., Kempermann, G. (1 Dec 2013). "Is silence golden? Effects of auditory stimuli and their absence on adult hippocampal neurogenesis." *Brain Structure & Function.*

14. Selhub, E., Logan, A. (2012). *Your brain on nature.* New York: Collins.

15. Correia, A. W., Peters, J. L., Levy, J. I., Melly, S., Dominici, F. (8 Oct 2013). "Residential exposure to aircraft noise and hospital admissions for cardiovascular diseases: Multi-airport retrospective study." *BMJ.* 347. doi: http://dx.doi.org/10.1136/bmj.f5561.

16. Klaus, F., Amrein, I. (14 Feb 2012). "Running in laboratory and wild rodents: Differences in context sensitivity and plasticity of hippocampal neurogenesis." *Behavioural Brain Research.* 227(2):363–70. doi: 10.1016/j.bbr.2011.04.027. Epub 27 Apr 2011.

17. Fujioka, A., Fujioka, T., Tsuruta, R., Izumi, T., Kasaoka, S., Maekawa, T. (13 Jan 2011). "Effects of a constant light environment on hippocampal neurogenesis and memory in mice." *Neuroscience Letters.* 488(1):41–4. doi: 10.1016/j.neulet.2010.11.001. Epub 5 Nov 2010.

18. Xie, L., Kang, H., Xu, Q., Chen, M., Liao, Y., Thiyagarajan, M., O'Donnell, J., Christensen, D. J., Nicholson, C., Iliff, J. J., Takano, T., Deane, R., Nedergaard, M. (18 Oct 2013). "Sleep drives metabolite clearance from the adult brain." *Science.* 342(6156):373–377. doi: 10.1126/science.1241224 REPORT.

19. (18 Nov 2013). *"The top 11 benefits of sex."* Mercola.com.

20. Marlatt, M. W., Potter, M. C., Lucassen, P. J., van Praag, H. (June 2012). "Running throughout middle-age improves memory function, hippocampal neurogenesis, and BDNF levels in female C57BL/6J mice." *Developmental Neurobiology.* 72(6):943–52. doi: 10.1002/dneu.22009.

21. Mustroph, M. L., Chen, S., Desai, S. C., Cay, E. B., DeYoung, E. K., Rhodes, J. S. (6 Sep 2012). "Aerobic exercise is the critical variable in an enriched environment that increases hippocampal neurogenesis and water maze learning in male

C57BL/6J mice." *Neuroscience.* 219:62–71. doi:10.1016/j. neuroscience.2012.06.007. Epub 12 Jun 2012.

22. Perlmutter, D. (2013). *Grain brain.* New York: Hachette Book Group, Inc.

23. Carter, C. S., and Porges, S. W. (Jan 2013). "Science and society: The biochemistry of love: An oxytocin hypothesis." *EMBO Report.* 14(1):12–16. doi: 10.1038/embor.2012.191. PMCID: PMC3537144. Epub 27 Nov 2012.

24. Glasper, E. R., Gould, E. (Apr 2013). "Sexual experience restores age-related decline in adult neurogenesis and hippocampal function." *Hippocampus.* 23(4):303–12. doi: 10.1002/hipo.22090. Epub 5 Mar 2013.

25. Fernandez, A., Goldberg, E., Michelon, P. (2013). *Sharp brains.* Seattle, WA: Amazon Digital Services.

26. Lehrer, J. (Feb-Mar, 2006) "The reinvention of the self." *Seed.*

27. Schmidt, A., et al. (19 March 2014). *Psychopharmacology.*

28. Ramírez-Rodríguez, G., Klempin, F., Babu, H., Benítez-King, G., Kempermann, G. (Aug 2009). "Melatonin modulates cell survival of new neurons in the hippocampus of adult mice." *Neuropsychopharmacology.* 34(9):2180–91. doi: 10.1038/npp.2009.46. Epub 6 May 2009.

29. Arden, J. (2014). *The brain bible.* New York: McGraw-Hill Education.

Heart

1. Siegal, D. (2012). *The developing mind.* 2nd Edition. New York: Guilford.

2. Pert, C. (2010). *Molecules of emotion.* New York: Simon and Schuster.

3. Cortright, B. (2007). *Integral psychology.* Albany, NY: SUNY Press.

4. Ekman, P. (2007). *The face of emotion."* 2nd Edition. New York: Holt.

5. Leasure, J. L., Decker, L. (2009). "Social isolation prevents exercise-induced proliferation of hippocampal progenitor cells in female rats." *Hippocampus.* 19:907–912.

6. Stranahan, A. M., Khalil, D., Gould, E. (2006). "Social isolation delays the positive effects of running on adult neurogenesis." *Nature Neuroscience.* 9:526–533.

7. Kozorovitskiy, Y., Gould, E. (2004). "Dominance hierarchy influences adult neurogenesis in the dentate gyrus." *Journal of Neuroscience.* 24:6755–6759.

8. McCormick, C. M., Thomas, C. M., Sheridan, C. S., Nixon, F., Flynn, J. A., et al. (2012). "Social instability stress in adolescent male rats alters hippocampal neurogenesis and produces deficits in spatial location memory in adulthood." *Hippocampus.* 22:1300–1312.

9. Leuner, B., Glasper, E. R., Gould, E. (2010). "Sexual experience promotes adult neurogenesis in the hippocampus despite an initial elevation in stress hormones." *PLoS One.* 5:e11597.

10. Leuner, B., Glasper, E. R., Gould, E. (2010). "Parenting and plasticity." *Trends in Neuroscience.* 33:465–473.

11. Glasper, E. R., Schoenfeld, T. J., Gould, E. (2012). "Adult neurogenesis: Optimizing hippocampal function to suit the environment." *Behavioural Brain Research.* 227:380–383.

12. Leuner, B., Mirescu, C., Noiman, L., Gould, E. (2007). "Maternal experience inhibits the production of immature neurons in the hippocampus during the postpartum period through elevations in adrenal steroids." *Hippocampus.* 17:434–442.

13. Mak, G. K., Weiss, S. (2010). "Paternal recognition of adult offspring mediated by newly generated CNS neurons." *Nature Neuroscience.* 13:753–758.

14. Corona, R., Larriva-Sahd, J., Paredes, R. G. (2011). "Paced-mating increases the number of adult new born cells in the internal cellular (granular) layer of the accessory olfactory bulb." *PLoS One.* 6(5):e19380.

15. Leuner, B., Glasper, E.R., Gould, E. (14 July 2010). "Sexual experience promotes adult neurogenesis in the hippocampus

despite an initial elevation in stress hormones." *PLoS One.* 5(7):e11597.

16. Oatridge, A., Holdcroft, A., Saeed, N., Hajnal, J. V., Puri, B. K., Fusi, L., Bydder, G. M. (Jan 2002). "Change in brain size during and after pregnancy: Study in healthy women and women with preeclampsia." *American Journal of Neuroradiology.* 23(1):19–26.

17. Galea, L. A., McEwen, B. S. (Mar 1999). "Sex and seasonal differences in the rate of cell proliferation in the dentate gyrus of adult wild meadow voles." *Neuroscience.* 89(3):955–64.

18. Lieberwirth, C.,* and Wang, Z. (2012). "The social environment and neurogenesis in the adult mammalian brain." *Frontiers in Human Neuroscience.* 6:118. doi: 10.3389/fnhum.2012.00118 PMCID: PMC3347626. Epub 8 May 2012.

19. Mak, G. K., Weiss, S. (2010). "Paternal recognition of adult offspring mediated by newly generated CNS neurons." *Nature Neuroscience.* 13:753–758. doi: 10.1038/nn.2550.

20. Steptoe, A. (1991). Invited review. "The links between stress and illness." *Journal of Psychosomatic. Research.* 35:633–644. doi: 10.1016/0022-3999(91)90113-3.

21. Curtis, R. (1995). "Stress, personality and illness: The move from generality to specificity in current research trends." *Irish Journal of Psychological Medicine.* 16:299–321.

22. Lieberwirth, C., Liu, Y., Jia, X., Wang, Z. (2012). "Social isolation impairs adult neurogenesis in the limbic system and alters behaviors in female prairie voles." *Hormones and Behavior.* doi: 10.1016/j.yhbeh.2012.03.005.

23. Goleman, D. (2006). *Social intelligence.* New York: Bantam.

24. Mitra, R., Sundlass, K., Parker, K. J., Schatzberg, A. F., Lyons, D. M. (2006). "Social stress-related behavior affects hippocampal cell proliferation in mice." *Physiology & Behavior.* 89:123–127. doi: 10.1016/j.physbeh.2006.05.047.

25. Yap, J. J., Takase, L. F., Kochman, L. J., Fornal, C. A., Miczek, K. A., Jacobs, B. L. (2006). "Repeated brief social defeat episodes in mice: Effects on cell proliferation in the dentate gyrus."

Behavioural Brain Research. 172:344–350. doi: 10.1016/j.bbr.2006.05.027

26. Kozorovitskiy, Y., Gould, E. (2004). "Dominance hierarchy influences adult neurogenesis in the dentate gyrus." *Journal of Neuroscience.* 24:6755–6759. doi: 10.1523/JNEUROSCI.0345-04.2004.

27. Sapolsky, R. (1998). *Why zebras don't get ulcers.* New York: Freeman and Company.

28. Barha, C. K., Lieblich, S. E., Galea, L. A. (2009). "Different forms of oestrogen rapidly upregulate cell proliferation in the dentate gyrus of adult female rats." *Journal of Neuroendocrinology.* 21:155–166. doi: 10.1111/j.1365-2826.2008.01809.x.

29. Spritzer, M. D., Galea, L. A. (2007). "Testosterone and dihydrotestosterone, but not estradiol, enhance survival of new hippocampal neurons in adult male rats." *Developmental Neurobiology.* 67:1321–1333. doi: 10.1002/dneu.20457.

30. Wong, E. Y., Herbert, J. (2005). "Roles of mineralocorticoid and glucocorticoid receptors in the regulation of progenitor proliferation in the adult hippocampus." *European Journal of Neuroscience.* 22:785–792. doi: 10.1111/j.1460-9568.2005.04277.x.

31. Tanapat, P., Hastings, N. B., Rydel, T. A., Galea, L. A., Gould, E. (2001). "Exposure to fox odor inhibits cell proliferation in the hippocampus of adult rats via an adrenal hormone-dependent mechanism." *Journal of Comparative Neurology.* 437:496–504. doi: 10.1002/cne.1297.

32. Leuner, B., Caponiti, J. M., Gould, E. (2012). "Oxytocin stimulates adult neurogenesis even under conditions of stress and elevated glucocorticoids." *Hippocampus.* 22:861–868. doi: 10.1002/hipo.20947.

33. Izard, C. E., & King, K. A. (2009). "Differential emotions theory." In K. Scherer (ed.), *Oxford Companion to the Affective Sciences.* 117–119. New York: Oxford University Press.

34. Mustroph, M. L., Chen, S., Desai, S. C., Cay, E. B., DeYoung, E. K., Rhodes, J. S.(6 Sep 2012). "Aerobic exercise is the critical variable in in an enriched environment that increases

hippocampal neurogenesis and water maze learning in male C57BL/6J mice" *Neuroscience.* 219:62–71. Epub 12 Jun 2012.

35. Roney, J. R., Lukaszwski, A. W., & Simmons, Z. L. (2007). "Rapid endocrine responses of young men to social interactions with young women." *Hormones and Behavior.* 52:326–333.

36. Roney, J. R., Simmons, Z. L., & Lukaszwski, A. W. (2010). "Androgen receptor gene sequence and basal cortisol concentrations predict men's hormonal response to potential mates." Proceedings of the Royal Society of London B. 277:57–63.

37. Roney, J. R. (2009). "The role of sex hormones in the initiation of human mating relationships." In P. T. Ellison & P. B. Gray (eds.), *The endocrinology of social relationships.* 246–269. Cambridge, MA: Harvard University Press.

38. Seligman, M. (2002). *Authentic happiness.* New York: Free Press.

39. Seligman, M. (2011). *Flourish.* New York: Free Press.

40. Hawkley, L. C., Thisted, R. A., Masi, C. M., and Cacioppo, J. T. (Mar 2010). "Loneliness predicts increased blood pressure: Five-year cross-lagged analyses in middle-aged and older adults." *Psychology and Aging.* 25(1):132–141. doi: 10.1037/a0017805.

41. Williams, R., & Williams, V. (1993). *Anger kills.* New York: HarperCollins.

42. Gage, F. (2011). "Interview with the Science Network." (12/11/2011) online.

43. Tindle, H. A., Chang, Y. F., Kuller, L. H., Manson, J. E., Robinson, J. G., Rosal, M. C., Siegle, G. J., Matthews, K. A. (25 Aug 2009). "Optimism, cynical hostility, and incident coronary heart disease and mortality in the Women's Health Initiative." *Circulation.* 120(8):656–62.

44. Tindle, H. A., Chang, Y. F., Kuller, L. H., Manson, J. E., Robinson, J. G., Rosal, M. C., Siegle, G. J., Matthews, K. A. (25 Aug 2009). "Optimism, cynical hostility, and incident coronary heart disease and mortality in the Women's Health Initiative." *Circulation.* 120(8):656–62.

45. Lund, R., Christensen, U., Juul Nilsson, C. Kriegbaum, M., Hulvej Rod, N. "Stressful social relations and mortality:

A prospective cohort study." *Journal of Epidemiology and Community Health.* doi:10.1136/jech-2013-203675.

46. Sapolsky, R. (1999). "Stress and your shrinking brain." *Discover.* 20(3):113–122.

47. Lu, L., Bao, G., Chen, H., Xia, P., Fan, X., Zhang, J., Pei, G., Ma, L. (Oct 2003). "Modification of hippocampal neurogenesis and neuroplasticity by social environments." *Experimental Neurology.* 183(2):600–9.

48. (2004). *Work, stress and health: The Whitehall II study.* London: Council of Civil Service Unions/ Cabinet Office.

49. Sapolsky, R. (1992). *Stress, the aging brain, and the mechanisms of neuron death.* Cambridge, MA: MIT Press.

50. Branon, N. (June-July 2007). "Stress kills brain cells off." *Scientific American.*

Mind

1. Reisberg, B. (Feb 1984). "Stages of cognitive decline." *American Journal of Nursing* (AJN). 84(2). From alz.org (Alzheimer's Association website).

2. Chertkow, H. (June 2002). "Mild cognitive impairment." *Canadian Alzheimer Disease Review.* 15–21.

3. Peterson, R. (Aug 2009). "Early diagnosis of Alzheimer's disease: Is MCI too late?" *Current Alzheimer Research.* 6(4):324–330.

4. Landau, S. M., Marks, S. M., Mormino, E. C., Rabinovici, G. D., Oh, H., O'Neil, J. P., Wilson, R. S., Jagust, W. J. (2012). "Association of lifetime cognitive engagement and low β-amyloid deposition." *Archives of Neurology.* doi: 10.1001/archneurol.2011.2748.

5. Fernandez, A., Goldberg, E., & Michelon, P. (2013). *"The sharpbrains guide to brain fitness."* National Science Foundation.

6. Wang, J. Y. J., Zhou, D. H. D., Li, J., Zhang, M., Deng, D. J., Tang, M., Gao, C., Li, J., Lian, Y., and Chen, M. (28 Mar

2006). "Leisure activity and risk of cognitive impairment: The Chongqing aging study." *Neurology.* 66(6):911–913.

7.   Melby-Lervag, M., and Hulme, C. (2012). "Is working memory training effective? A meta-analytic review." *Developmental Psychology.* doi: 10.1037/a0028228.

8.   Ericcson, K. A., Chase, W. G., Faloon, S. (June 1980). "Acquisition of a memory skill." *Science.* 208(4448):1181–2. doi: 10.1126/science.7375930. PMID 7375930.

9.   Conway, A. R., Kane, M. J., Engle, R. W. (Dec 2003). "Working memory capacity and its relation to general intelligence." *Trends in Cognitive Science (Regular Edition).* 7(12):547–52. doi: 10.1016/j.tics.2003.10.005. PMID 14643371.

10. Gould, E., Beylin, A., Tanapat, P., Reeves, A., Shors, T. (1999). "Learning enhances adult neurogenesis in the hippocampal formation." *Nature Neuroscience.* 2:260–5.

Spirit

1.   Smith, H. (1992). *Forgotten truth.* New York: HarperOne.

2.   Kabat-Zinn, J. (1990). *Full catastrophe living.* New York: Delta.

3.   Kabat-Zinn, J. (2005). *Wherever you go, there you are.* New York: Hyperion.

4.   MacDonald, D., Walsh, R., Shapiro, S. (2013). "Meditation" chapter. In *The Wiley-Blackwell handbook of transpersonal psychology.* Friedman & Hartelius (eds.) West Sussex, UK: Wiley-Blackwell.

5.   Williams, M., Teasdale, J, Segal, Z., Kabat-Zin, J. (2012). *The mindful way through depression.* New York: Guilford Press.

6.   Robinson, P., & Strosahl, K. (2008). *The mindfulness and acceptance workbook for depression.* Oakland: New Harbinger.

7.   Luders, E., Thompson, P. M., Kurth, F., Hong, J. Y., Phillips, O. R., Wang, Y., Gutman, B. A., Chou, Y. Y., Narr, K. L., Toga, A. W. (Dec 2013). "Global and regional alterations of hippocampal anatomy in long-term meditation practitioners." *Human Brain*

Mapping. 34(12):3369–75. doi: 10.1002/hbm.22153. Epub 19 Jul 2012.

8. Hölzel, B. K., Carmody, J., Vangel, M., Congleton, C., Yerramsetti, S. M., Gard, T., Lazar, S. W. (30 Jan 2011). "Mindfulness practice leads to increases in regional brain gray matter density." *Psychiatry Research Journal.* 191(1):36–43. doi: 10.1016/j.pscychresns.2010.08.006. Epub 10 Nov 2010.

9. Monti, D. A., Kash, K. M., Kunkel, E. J., Brainard, G., Wintering, N., Moss, A. S., Rao, H., Zhu, S., Newberg, A. B. (Dec 2012). "Changes in cerebral blood flow and anxiety associated with an 8-week mindfulness programme in women with breast cancer." *Stress Health.* 28(5):397–407. doi: 10.1002/smi.2470.

10. Leung, M. K., Chan, C. C., Yin, J., Lee, C. F., So, K. F., Lee, T. M. (18 July 2013). "Increased gray matter volume in the right angular and posterior parahippocampal gyri in loving-kindness meditators." *Social Cognitive and Affective Neuroscience.* 8(1):34–9. doi: 10.1093/scan/nss076. Epub 18 Jul 2012.

11. Hofmann, S. G., Grossman, P., Hinton, D. E. (Nov 2011). "Loving-kindness and compassion meditation: Potential for psychological interventions." *Clinical Psychology Review.* 31(7):1126–32. doi: 10.1016/j.cpr.2011.07.003. Epub 26 Jul 2011.

12. Childre, D. & Martin, H. (1990). *The heartmath solution.* New York: HarperCollins Publishers.

13. Luders, E.,* Kurth, F., Toga, A. W., Narr, K. L., and Gaser, C. "Meditation effects within the hippocampal complex revealed by voxel-based morphometry and cytoarchitectonic probabilistic mapping." *Frontiers in Psychology.* Epub 9 Jul 2013.

14. Hölzel, B. K., Ott, U., Gard, T., Hempel, H., Weygandt, M., Morgen, K., Vaitl, D. (Mar 2008). "Investigation of mindfulness meditation practitioners with voxel-based morphometry." *Social Cognitive and Affective Neuroscience.* 3(1):55–61.

15. Luders, E., Toga, A. W., Lepore, N., Gaser, C. (15 Apr 2009). "The underlying anatomical correlates of long-term meditation: Larger hippocampal and frontal volumes of gray matter." *Neuroimage.* 45(3):6728.

16. Luders, E., Clark, K., Narr, K. L., Toga, A. W. (15 Aug 2011). "Enhanced brain connectivity in long-term meditation practitioners." *Neuroimage.* 57(4):1308–16.

17. Luders, E., Thompson, P. M., Kurth, F., Hong, J. Y., Phillips, O. R., Wang, Y., Gutman, B. A., Chou, Y. Y., Narr, K. L., Toga, A. W. (Dec 2013). "Global and regional alterations of hippocampal anatomy in long-term meditation practitioners." *Human Brain Mapping.* 34(12):3369–75.

18. Murakami H., Nakao, T., Matsunaga, M., Kasuya, Y., Shinoda, J., Yamada, J., Ohira, H. (2012). "The structure of mindful brain." *PLoS One.* 7(9):e46377.

19. Leung, M. K., Chan, C. C., Yin, J., Lee, C. F., So, K. F., Lee, T. M. (Jan 2013). "Increased gray matter volume in the right angular and posterior parahippocampal gyri in loving-kindness meditators." *Social Cognitive and Affective Neuroscience.* 8(1):34–9.

20. Williams, J. M., Teasdale, J. D., Segal, Z. V., Soulsby, J. (Feb 2000). "Mindfulness-based cognitive therapy reduces overgeneral autobiographical memory in formerly depressed patients." *Journal of Abnormal Psychology.* 109(1):150–5.

21. Heeren, A., Van Broeck, N., Philippot, P. (May 2009). "The effects of mindfulness on executive processes and autobiographical memory specificity." *Behaviour Research and Therapy.* 47(5):403–9.

22. Kozhevnikov, M., Louchakova, O., Josipovic, Z., Motes, M. A. (May 2009). "The enhancement of visuospatial processing efficiency through Buddhist Deity meditation." *Psychological Science.* 20(5):645–53.

23. Chiesa, A., Calati, R., Serretti, A. (Apr 2011). "Does mindfulness training improve cognitive abilities? A systematic review of neuropsychological findings." *Clinical Psychological Review.* 31(3):449–64.

24. Tooley, G. A., Armstrong, S. M., Norman, T. R., Sali, A. (May 2000). "Acute increases in night-time plasma melatonin levels following a period of meditation." *Biological Psychology.* 53(1):69–78.

25. Pace, T. W. W., Tenzin Negi, L., Adame, D. D., Cole, S. P., Sivilli, T. I., Brown, T. D., Issa, M. J., Raison, C. L.,* Effect of compassion meditation on neuroendocrine, innate immune and behavioral responses to psychosocial stress." *Psychoneuroendocrinology.* 34:87–98.

26. Benson, H. (2000). *The relaxation response.* New York: HarperTorch.

27. Solberg, E. E., Holen, A., Ekeberg, Ø., Østerud, B., Halvorsen, R., Sandvik, L. (Mar 2004). "The effects of long meditation on plasma melatonin and blood serotonin." *Medical Science Monitor.* doi: 10(3):CR96–101. Epub 1 Mar 2004.

28. Walsh, R. (1991). *The spirit of shamanism.* Los Angeles: Tarcher.

Increase Neurogenesis by Not Slowing It Down

1. Centers for Disease Control and Prevention. (2011). FASTSTATS – "Leading Causes of Death." cdc.gov. 2011; Available at: http://www.cdc.gov/NCHS/fastats/Default.htm

2. Bastard, J. P., Maachi, M., Lagathu, C., et al. (2006). "Recent advances in the relationship between obesity, inflammation, and insulin resistance." *European Cytokine Network.* 17(1):4–12.

3. Cao, J. J. (2011). "Effects of obesity on bone metabolism." *Journal of Orthopaedic Surgery and Research.* 6:30.

4. Jha, R. K., Ma, Q., Sha, H., and Palikhe, M. (2009). "Acute pancreatitis: A literature review." *Medical Science Monitor.* 15(7):RA147–56.

5. Ferrucci, L., Semba, R. D., Guralnik, J. M., et al. (2010). "Proinflammatory state, hepcidin, and anemia in older persons." *Blood.* 115(18):3810–3816.

6. Glorieux, G., Cohen, G., Jankowski, J., and Vanholder, R. (2009). "Platelet/leukocyte activation, inflammation, and uremia." *Seminars in Dialysis.* 22(4):423–427

7. Kundu, J. K., and Surh, Y. J. (2008). "Inflammation: Gearing the journey to cancer." *Mutation Research.* 659(1-2):15–30.

8. Murphy, S. L., et al. "Deaths: Preliminary Data for 2010." *National Vital Statistics Report.* 60:4. (1/11/2012).

9. Singh, T., and Newman, A. B. (2011). "Inflammatory markers in population studies of aging." *Ageing Research Review.* 10(3):319–329.

10. Pompl, P. N., et al. (2003). "A therapeutic role for cyclooxygenase-2 inhibitors in a transgenic mouse model of amyotrophic lateral sclerosis." *FASEB Journal.* doi: 10.1096/fj.02-0876fje.

11. Teismann, P., et al. (2003). "Cyclooxygenase-2 is instrumental in Parkinson's disease neurodegeneration." *PNAS.* 100(9):5473–5478.

12. Karin, M., Lawrence, T., and Nizet, V. (2006). "Innate immunity gone awry: Linking microbial infections to chronic inflammation and cancer." *Cell.* 124(4):823–835.

13. Klegeris, A., et al. (2002). "Cyclooxygenase and 5 lipooxygenase inhibitors protect against mononuclear phagocyte neurotoxicity." *Neurobiology of Aging.* (23)787–794.

14. Jorm, A. F., et al. (1987). "The prevalence of dementia: A quantitative integration of the literature." *Acta Psychiatrica Scandinavica.* 76:465–479.

15. Bremmer, J. D. (1999). "Does stress damage the brain?" *Biological Psychiatry.* 45:797–805.

16. Gurvits, T. G., Shenton, M. R., Hokama, H., et al. (1989). "Magnetic resonance imaging study of hippocampal volume in chronic combat-related posttraumatic stress disorder." *Biological Psychiatry.* 40:192–199.

17. Gurvits, T. G., Lasko, N. B., Schacter, S. C., Kuhne, A. A., Orr, S. P., Pitman, R. K. (1993). "Neurological status of Vietnam veterans with chronic posttraumatic stress disorder." *Journal of Neuropsychiatry and Clinical Neurosciences.* 5:183–188.

18. Sapolsky, R. (1999). "Stress and your shrinking brain." *Discover.* 20(3), 113–122.

19. Yandoli, K. (2013). "Teens and stress." Huffington Post. (2/12/2013).

20. (1 Apr 2013). "Men Are From Mars." *Science Daily.* sciencedaily.com.

21. Kaler, S. R., Freeman, B. J. (May 1994). "Analysis of environmental deprivation: Cognitive and social development in Romanian orphans." *Journal of Child Psychology and Psychiatry.* 35(4):769–81. doi: 10.1111/j.1469-7610.1994.tb01220.x. PMID 7518826.

22. Rutter, M., Andersen-Wood, L., Beckett, C., et al. (May 1999). "Quasi-autistic patterns following severe early global privation. English and Romanian adoptees (ERA) study team." *Journal of Child Psychology and Psychiatry.* 40(4):537–49. doi: 10.1017/S0021963099003935. PMID 10357161.

23. Windsor, J., Glaze, L. E., Koga, S. F. (Oct 2007). "Language acquisition with limited input: Romanian institution and foster care." *Journal of Speech Language and Hearing Research.* 50(5):1365–81. doi: 10.1044/1092-4388(2007/095). PMID 17905917.

24. Beckett, C., Maughan, B., Rutter, M., et al. (2006). "Do the effects of early severe deprivation on cognition persist into early adolescence? Findings from the English and Romanian adoptees study." *Child Development.* 77(3):696–711. doi: 10.1111/j.1467-8624.2006.00898.x. PMID 16686796.

25. Chugani, H. T., Behen, M. E., Muzik, O., Juhász, C., Nagy, F., Chugani, D. C. (Dec 2001). "Local brain functional activity following early deprivation: A study of postinstitutionalized Romanian orphans." *Neuroimage.* 14(6):1290–301. doi: 10.1006/nimg.2001.0917. PMID 11707085.

26. Fan, Y., Liu, Z., Weinstein, P. R., Fike, J. R., Liu, J. (Jan 2007). "Environmental enrichment enhances neurogenesis and improves functional outcome after cranial irradiation." *European Journal of Neuroscience.* 25(1):38–46. doi: 10.1111/j.1460-9568.2006.05269.x. PMID 17241265.

27. Diamond, M. C., Krech, D., Rosenzweig, M. R. (Aug 1964). "The effects of an enriched environment on the histology of the rat cerebral cortex." *Journal of Comparative. Neurology.* 123:111–20. doi: 10.1002/cne.901230110. PMID 14199261.

28. Diamond, M. C., Law, F., Rhodes, H., et al. (Sep 1966). "Increases in cortical depth and glia numbers in rats subjected

to enriched environment." *Journal of Comparative Neurology.* 128(1):117–26. doi: 10.1002/cne.901280110. PMID 4165855.

29. Greenough, W. T., Volkmar, F. R. (Aug 1973). "Pattern of dendritic branching in occipital cortex of rats reared in complex environments." *Experimental Neurology.* 40(2):491–504. doi: 10.1016/0014-4886(73)90090-3. PMID 4730268.

30. Volkmar, F. R., Greenough, W. T. (June 1972). "Rearing complexity affects branching of dendrites in the visual cortex of the rat." *Science.* 176 (4042):1445–7. doi: 10.1126/science.176.4042.1445. PMID 5033647.

31. Borowsky, I. W., Collins, R. C. (Oct 1989). "Metabolic anatomy of brain: A comparison of regional capillary density, glucose metabolism, and enzyme activities." *Journal of Comparative Neurology.* 288(3):401–13. doi: 10.1002/cne.902880304. PMID 2551935.

32. Sirevaag, A. M., Greenough, W. T. (Oct 1987). "Differential rearing effects on rat visual cortex synapses. III. Neuronal and glial nuclei, boutons, dendrites, and capillaries." *Brain Research.* 424(2):320–32. doi: 10.1016/0006-8993(87)91477-6. PMID 3676831.

33. Cohen, S., Janicki-Deverts, D., Doyle, W. J., Miller, G. E., Frank, E., Rabin, B. S., and Turner, R. B. (2 Apr 2012). "Chronic stress, glucocorticoid receptor resistance, inflammation, and disease risk." *PNAS.* doi: 10.1073/pnas.1118355109.

34. UCSF News, July 19, 2011.

35. (May 2014). "Long-term cumulative depressive symptom burden and risk of cognitive decline and dementia among very old women." *Journals of Gerontology: Series A: Biological Sciences and Medical Science.* 69(5):595–601. doi: 10.1093/gerona/glt139. Epub 4 Oct 2013.

36. Zeki, A., Hazzouri, A., Vittinghoff, E., Byers, A., Covinsky, K., Blazer, D., Diem, S., Ensrud, K. E., Yaffe K. (2014) Research report: "Stressful social relations and mortality: A prospective cohort study." *Journal of Epidemiology and Community Health.* doi: 10.1136/jech-2013-203675.

37. Lund, R., Christensen, U., Juul Nilsson, C., Kriegbaum, M., Hulvej Rod, N. (Feb 2013). "Adverse oral health and cognitive decline: The health, aging and body composition study." *Journal of the American Geriatrics Society*. 61(2):177–84. doi: 10.1111/jgs.12094.

38. Stewart, R., Weyant, R. J., Garcia, M. E., Harris, T., Launer, L. J., Satterfield, S., Simonsick, E. M., Yaffe, K., Newman, A. B. (Jan 2012). "C-reactive protein is related to memory and medial temporal brain volume in older adults." *Brain, Behavior, and Immunity*. 26(1):103–8. doi: 10.1016/j.bbi.2011.07.240. Epub 6 Aug 2011.

39. Sapolsky, R. M., Uno, H., Rebert, C. S., and Finch, C. E. (1990). "Hippocampal damage associated with prolonged glucocorticoid exposure in primates." *Journal of Neuroscience*. 10(9): 2897–290.

40. Cohen, S., et al. (2 Apr 2012). "Chronic stress, glucocorticoid receptor resistance, inflammation, and disease risk." *PNAS*.

Putting It All Together

1. Kempermann, G., Gast, D., Gage, F. H. (Aug 2002). "Neuroplasticity in old age: Sustained fivefold induction of hippocampal neurogenesis by long-term environmental enrichment." *Annals of Neurology*. 52(2):135–43.

Appendix A

1. MacLean, P. (1990). *The triune brain in evolution*. Springer: New York.

2. Pearce, J. (2004). "Nurturance: A biological imperative." *Shift*. 3: 16–19.

3. Amen, D. (2012). *Use your brain to change your age*. Crown Archetype: New York.

4. Siegel, D. (2001). *The developing mind*. Guilford: New York.

5. Schore, A. (2003). *Affect regulation and the repair of the self*. W. W. Norton & Co.: New York.

6. Siegel, D. (2010). *The mindful therapist.* W. W. Norton & Co.: New York.

7. Gage, F. (Aug 2000). "Reinventing the brain." *Life Extension Magazine* interview.

8. Lewis, T., Amini, F., Lannon, R. (2000). *A general theory of love.* New York: Random House

9. Arden, J. (2014). *The brain bible.* New York: McGraw-Hill Education.

10. Fernandez, A., Goldberg, E., & Michelon, P. (2013). *The sharpbrains guide to brain fitness.* National Science Foundation.

11. Ekman, P. (2007). *The face of emotion.* 2nd Edition. New York: Holt.

12. Sapolsky, R. (1999). "Stress and your shrinking brain." *Discover.* 20(3):116–122.

13. Tanti, A., et al. (2011). "Region-specific regulation of neurogenesis along the septo-temporal axis of the hippocampus by stress, antidepressants and environmental enrichment." *Neuroscience.* (Poster session 11/13/2011).

ACKNOWLEDGEMENTS

I am deeply grateful to many people who helped bring this book into existence. Mytrae Meliana has been unfailingly supportive throughout many weekends and days spent writing, as well as a helpful critic and editor. Philip Brooks read an early draft and gave invaluable comments that helped both content and style. Cathy Coleman's feedback aided in shaping this book's eventual form. Virginia Kahn provided key suggestions at different times of the writing. Rick Cortright gave copyediting feedback at an early stage that was extremely helpful. Cary Hammer's feedback and suggestions on the first chapter were gifts from editorial heaven.

Jeff Shapiro gave meticulous feedback on the first part, and Paul Linn provided big picture support and critical feedback that helped move the writing forward. My copyeditor, Madeline Hopkins, has an eagle eye for spotting tiny errors as well as a clarifying sense that improved the first chapters especially.

My psychotherapy clients have been wonderful teachers and have reinforced for me how important healthy brain function is in optimal functioning. They have demonstrated that brain healthy living involves every level of being: body, heart, mind, spirit.

ABOUT THE AUTHOR

Brant Cortright, Ph.D., is a clinical psychologist and Professor of Psychology at California Institute of Integral Studies. His consulting practice specializes in cutting-edge brain health and neuroscience-informed depth therapy. He is the author of two other books, Psychotherapy and Spirit as well as Integral Psychology (both published by SUNY Press.) He currently lives in the San Francisco Bay Area.

Visit him on the web at: www//brantcortright.com.

If you enjoyed this book please consider writing a review on Amazon.